To:
Sacramento
Center
From: A.K. Buckroth and
Be Happy! Be Healthy and
Take Care!

MY DIABETIC SOUL

An Autobiography

By A. K. Buckroth

Published by
PRISMATIC PUBLISHING
1000 Sunrise Ave. Ste. 9B Box 310
Roseville, CA 95661

Official Paperback Edition

Published by Prismatic Publishing
1000 Sunrise Ave Ste 9B Box 310
Roseville, CA 95661

Distributed by Simplie Indie, a Division of Prismatic Entertainment, Inc.
www.SimplieIndie.com

www.MyDiabeticSoul.com
www.Buckroth.Wordpress.com

ISBN-13: 978-0-9822030-9-5
ISBN- 10: 0-9822030-9-8

First Edition: February 2010

Cover layout and design by Bill Walker

DISCLAIMER

As an author, A. K. Buckroth has made efforts to embellish her opinions with facts of research – either through, and not limited to, internet research, book readings, newspaper and magazine articles - hoping to ensure up-to-date accuracy with awareness for all readers. She assumes no responsibility for errors, accuracies or inaccuracies, omissions, or inconsistencies. Any misgivings against people and/or organizations are unintentional. Readers are encouraged to research for facts.

Names have not been changed to protect the innocent or the guilty.

While the author/publisher have used best efforts in preparing this book, no representations or warranties have been made with respect to the accuracy or completeness of the contents of this book and specifically disclaim any implied warranties of merchantability or fitness for a particular purpose. No warranty may be created or extended by sales representatives or written sales materials. The advice and strategies contained herein may not be suitable for your situation. You should consult with a professional where and when appropriate. The author/publisher shall not be liable for any loss of profit or any other commercial damages, including but not limited to special, incidental, consequential, or other damages.

It is the authors' intent to donate a percentage of the selling profits of this book for the ongoing care, inspiration, encouragement, and teaching capabilities to **The Barton Center for Diabetes Education, Inc., P. O. Box 356, North Oxford, Massachusetts, 01537**.

Theirs is a historical and continual light of hope!

Acknowledgments

Grateful for his immediate trouble-shooting skills, his computer knowledge and his uncanny and split-second ability to come up what I need, my husband, Wayne, has been ever-present throughout this project. Thanks to my childhood friend, Ricky Wołosz, for his witty yet sarcastic memories of the times we spent together in elementary and high schools. Thank yous to my friend, Tamara Dorris, for her ability to lead me to where I needed to be in order to learn on my own without her giving me specific details. Her actions reminded me of leading a horse to water but not being able to make it drink. That just would have been too easy! Debby Shallenberger for her *Daily Inspirations*. They helped – a lot. Thank you to the many acquaintances I have met during the Sacramento [California] Suburban Writers Club. Their experiences and knowledge individually and together helped encourage this work of art. Jerry Kennedy for guiding and guarding me through the endless realm of virtual marketing. Bill Walker for insurmountable skills in putting this all together.

To my mother,
Theresa Viola,
whose prayers alone
have given me a continuous onslaught of hope,
especially when hope is forgotten.

Table of Contents

INTRODUCTION

Accomplishing a first marathon is an extremely proud and momentous occasion especially when training takes nine months before the actual event. This was my first marathon through the American Diabetes Association (ADA). Having been in existence for the last twenty-five years or so, personal familiarity with this organization was all too comfortable. I am one of three diabetics in a family of five biological children.

With a deep personal interest involved, such an affair became all encompassing. Having raised $2,000.00 of the required $3,000.00, I was proudly on my way to Dublin, Ireland, to take part in that country's "Friendly Marathon."

And so it was. After completing a little more than half the marathon, 17 miles to be exact, I decided to be a tourist and enjoy the rest of the scenery with my husband before my knees wore out completely. But this book is not about that beautiful country or my glorious touristy adventures. It is about me. This is my story. I was diagnosed with diabetes in 1959 at the precious age of 2. At this writing I have been diabetic for fifty years. I almost gladly entitled this work *Diabetes: Infancy to Menopause*, but the present name came about through a particular fact that you will read on page 34. Yes, I honestly believe I was born with *it*. *It* didn't "just happen," and then was diagnosed a few years later.

In the meantime, many other books, articles (some written by me), magazine publications, etc., on the subject of diabetes are in existence and have been throughout my life. Media attention granted to this subject brings a trickle of joy to my soul if only to think that people are thinking about *it*.

This disease, already known as an "epidemic," has in recent years been labeled as a "pandemic." This means that *it* now covers and concerns the world and has become a frightening fact. It frightens me. Simply, it is "out of control," a huge degradation for the

1

diabetics that fight to survive, that fight to keep their bodies in one piece, that fight to sustain jobs, careers, family and overall happiness. A diabetic like me. Sadly enough, the continuous fundraising for more and more research has become a bottomless pit.

"Write a book!" bellowed Owen while driving the tour bus. "Write. Write it down. All of it, no matter what it is!" Therefore, I share the story of my life with diabetes with you. Having written it has been a dream come true.

After completion of this marathon and my two-week stay in Ireland, the 'bellowing' bus driver, Owen, became a brief yet essential character in my life at that time. It is proof to me of how all of humanity is linked in one continuous chain. It was during a tour through northwestern Ireland, its coast and inlay, that Owen proclaimed his thoughts. Owen is an inspiration to this writing.

My endeavors, all of them specifically for this particular event – the nine-months of training, the time, the diet, the wardrobe, the taping of feet, special attention to footwear, and more time – were for the cure of this baffling and devastating disease known as *Diabetes*. After all, having been medically classified as a "juvenile diabetic," that is what I was to remain all my life. Then again, maybe not. Maybe I will be given a shot to make this go away! That title, *Juvenile Diabetic*, also became a learned stereotype on me in the medical community.

My siblings and I have knocked door-to-door for monetary contributions for a cure toward diabetes when we were children. That experience is explained on page 51. Also having participated in yearly 5k and 10k walks to raise money toward the cure has culminated over the last four and a half decades of my life. This particular marathon was to be special. Although I have not limited my fundraising activities to diabetes, I have "wogged" for other fundraisers (e.g., Multiple Sclerosis, Heart Disease, Lung Disease, Breast Cancer, Leukemia, etc).

"Wogging" is a phrase I like to claim fame to: it is the act of walking and jogging. There's also "wog-run" where I have started off running, going into a speedier jog if only because I feel good, knowing I can continue for another minute and then break out in a sweaty yet exhilarating run; slow down to a jog and back to a brisk walk. Once mentioning this to others, I am looked at quizzically and asked for an explanation. The term has since come to my ears from the lips of others. That makes me smile. Creativity always at play! *It* was understood meaning *I* was understood.

The highlight of *this* particular marathon was again for *the* cure, the actual cure of diabetes. I believed it was going to happen if only because I was a part of this team – this team of strangers that were also walking, wogging, running people who believed along with me. Well, knowing that personal participation was a necessity - a dire necessity - I was ready, willing, able, and determined to assist with the cure for this uncomfortably progressive disease. Anticipation was overflowing! Sponsors were continually contacted and updated; sponsorship checks were rolling in to help fulfill a *required* commitment to meet the ADA's goal per participant at $3.000.00. My energy level was overflowing!

Family, friends, neighbors, strangers believed along with me. I had their checks, I had their cash. They were all going to help me wog and get that cure! I felt blessed.

Scheduled to take place on October 30, 2000, this "Friendly Marathon" brought a delightful, anticipatory visit to Ireland. Never having visited this part of Europe, excitement was enhanced through the overall participation of this marathon and my having made a *huge* commitment. With that monetary goal figure in mind along with the registration fee, the personal training, and the bulk of tremendous planning and organizing, February was a great time to start! When September rolled around and I accomplished 17.5 miles along the concrete shore of the Pacific Ocean in 3.5 hours between the cities of Torrance, California, and Manhattan Beach, California, I knew I was ready. Self-perseverance with a positive attitude became one and the same. This attitude was grown and nurtured from my very beginnings! I knew what my body could and could not take. Once again I was learning and re-learning how to take care of myself.

With a diligent and purposefully pre-planned earlier arrival than was expected to Ireland, departure took place from Los Angeles International Airport (LAX) on October 25th to arrive in Dublin International Airport (DUB) on October 26th. As the marathon schedule was to take place on October 30th, this early-bird planning was for good reason. I needed to adjust my insulin dosages, get acquainted and acclimated with the environment, learn where available restaurants and foods stores were, as well as become psychologically ready for this endeavor.

I must tell you, I wasn't alone. My husband of ten years at the time, Wayne, rented a bicycle when we reached Dublin, Ireland, and was able to ride by my side as I wogged. As it was bitter cold and rainy, known as the "worst storm in fifty years," Wayne wore socks on his hands because of no available gloves. We were not expecting and not prepared for such miserably wet and cold weather. On his back he toted a backpack full of water, juices, granola bars, peanut butter crackers, and glucose tabs – just in case. I am ever so glad he did because there were no such preparations that I saw on our route. He carried enough for a few other marathoners if the need arose. Many of them are diabetics.

And so, dear reader, I've walked in your shoes, *wogged* in your shoes, and maybe even ran in them! I consider this book as a deadline to my life. I must share my story, my life as a diabetic, with you who know all too well or do not know at all. If you believe as I do, my intuition, my spirit, my soul has been energized to write this book. I want to be an inspiration for you. There has not been a day or night in the many years that it took to accomplish this task that my conscious mind, through angelic voices or spirit guides, has encouraged and motivated this effort. Yes, this dream has been side-tracked. However, I need to be of service to you, dear reader, through this story of my life with diabetes.

Be aware that, even though this is an autobiography, much research is used to express facts with my personal opinions.

I describe myself as being a winsome, attractive, extremely

personable, knowledgeable, resourceful, and helpful woman; a 'giver' as opposed to a 'taker. In no way, shape or form does my physique even hint at the terminal condition that assails my body.

I am a realist, I am an optimist, I am a believer, I am always a learner, I am many things. I invite you to encounter my life. I need you to know what is has been like.

My life has been a tapestry
Of rich and royal hue.
An everlasting vision
Of an ever-changing view.
A wondrous woven magic
In bits of blue and gold.
A tapestry to feel and see,
Impossible to hold.
Once amid the soft
Silver sadness in the sky,
There came a man of fortune-
A drifter passing by.
He wore a torn and tattered cloth
Around his leathered hide
And a coat of many colors,
Yellow green on either side.
He moved with some uncertainty
As if he didn't know
Just what he was there for
Or where he ought to go.
Once he reached for something
Golden hanging from a tree
But his hand came down empty.
Soon within my tapestry
Along the rutted road
He sat down on a river rock
And turned in to a toad.
It seemed that he had fallen

My Diabetic Soul

Into someone's wicked spell.
And I wept to see him suffer,
Though I didn't know him well.
As I watched in sorrow
There suddenly appeared
A figure grey and ghostly
Beneath a flowing beard.
In times of deepest darkness
I've seen him dressed in black.
Now my tapestry's unraveling.
He's come to take me back.
He's come to take me back.

Sung by Carole King on her "Tapestry" Album/CD.

Chapter 1
Origins

The era was the 1950's. A happy time, a rockin' and rollin' time. Although I was born later in the decade, the mood lingered.

Front page news headlines displayed such titles as: *"President Eisenhower Sworn Into Office for Second Term;" "Eisenhower signs Civil Rights Act of 1957;" "USSR Sends Sputnik into Space;"* and *"Interferon is discovered."*

Do *you* remember this stuff? I don't.

How about trends of poodle haircuts, black and white saddle shoes, Silly Putty, and Hula Hoops? *Althea Gibson* was the first African-American woman to win the U. S. Open tennis title, while *Don Bowden* was the first U. S. runner to break the 4-minute mile.

Top tunes were: *"A White Sport Coat and a Pink Carnation," "All Shook Up," "Jailhouse Rock," "Lucille,"* and *"Love Letters in the Sand."* The most popular television shows, in black-and-white, were *"Wagon Train," "Maverick," "Leave it to Beaver,"* and *"Perry Mason."* Movie stars such as Jerry Lewis, Rock Hudson, John Wayne, Elvis Presley, and Yul Brynner were the cat's meow. Jerry Lewis still is!

Furthermore, it was in 1957 that New York loses Giants and Dodgers to California; *"The Music Man"* opened on Broadway; DNA is synthesized; drive-in movie theaters peaked to popularity, a new Ford cost $2,045.00; and factory workers earned $2.00 an hour. All here in the good 'ol United States!

No, I don't remember *all* these facts. The ones I do remember were always shared while my mother was present, usually while she ironed as the black and white television played.

My Diabetic Soul

Born to a United States Naval Chief and a promising fashion designer/seamstress in Portsmouth, Virginia, my mother gave up her career to concentrate on the specialties needed to assist her second of three children at the time. The year was 1957 and the U. S. Navy needed my father to concentrate on his assignments, always leaving his young wife to care for their children, alone, for weeks on end.

As thinly related to me, my father was born to German immigrants. It wasn't until the mid-nineteen eighties that I learned from my father's elderly cousins whom emigrated to Canada that Estonia was the paternal family's country of origin. With the ensuing communist controversy at that time, it seems that the country of Estonia was back-and-forth trying to maintain its own identity while being subject to the captive auspices of Germany. These specific cousins literally and physically ran away from the horrors that took place in the early 20th century.

I recall being told that my father's father was a Lutheran Minister who captivated audiences in Boston Common. His name was Frederick Buchroth. I know even less about his mother, my paternal Grandmother, Lydia, other than the sketchy fact that they resided in Hyde Park, Massachusetts, after a move from Chicago, Illinois. That is where my father was born. No one was available to embellish or encourage this ancestry. My paternal genealogy never went much farther than that and my imagination. However, Lydia re-married a wonderful man by the name of John Underhill, who became known to me and my siblings as *dziadzi* (short for *dziadek),* Polish for *Grandfather.*

My mother, however, was the fifth child of six siblings born to Polish immigrants. Her demeanor remains strong, full-proof, and *very* Catholic which seems to be typical of that ethnicity.

After their sojourn to the United States via the infamous *Ellis Island,* New York State, my maternal grandparents, Mary and Alexander, were greeted a new beginning also in the very early 19th century. From what I am to understand, this couple met in Massachusetts, married, toiled New England, raised six children, and died.

You'll become somewhat acquainted with my Polish/American upbringing as this story continues.

As told to me years later, mom was in tears too often due to my sickness. That's the way it was: father breadwinner through the government; mother caretaker and housewife; children 'Navy brats'. Not glamorous by any means, diabetes requires change and extra monetary allotments, often at the expense of tangibles as well as intangibles. As all couples of the time, my parents did what they had to do, what they could. They were one couple among thousands embedded in the income status as "military poor." Stationed in Portsmouth, Norfolk County, Virginia at the time, our humble trailer home was filled with five: two parents and three children. My brother, Charles, was born then and there as well. As told to me many years later by my father, a Navy Chief, I was named after the glamorous ocean liner, the "Andrea Doria." It seems perfectly befitting my life. A short story follows:

"It was Wednesday, July 25th 1956. At 11:10pm on a dark and foggy night, two great ocean liners, *T/N Andrea Doria* and *MV Stockholm*, collided near Nantucket, Massachusetts. I was there, I am a survivor…My name is Anthony Grillo…"
(**www.AndreaDoria.org**.)

After seeing the movie "*The Perfect Storm*" numerous times, I can't help but wonder if there are any *Andrea Gail's* out there. It's a New England thing.

This diabetes diagnosis in 1959 was due to Mom's suspicions of my daily activities. With a surge of energy to climb the kitchen counter, invading the cookie jar, followed with an *immense* thirst for anything drinkable, to napping wherever and whenever led her to bring me to the Naval Hospital's Emergency Room. Hospitalized for seven days, I lapsed into a coma for approximately 24 hours. I just must have been exhausted! All that climbing, you know.

I can only imagine my parents' anguish. I was 2 years old. What did I know? What did they know? I certainly have no recollections of my first insulin injections; or my first use of Clinitest tablets for glucose urine testing at that time; nor scheduled and "balanced" meal planning; nor the tears my mother shed in her attempts to keep her baby healthy and alive. I can only imagine the heartbreak and fright. "Where did this come from? How did my daughter get this?" she would continually ask many physicians.

Many of you, dear readers, know the same. On and on and on. To this day, those questions continue unanswered. Too many theories have been born.

I grew up with the speculation that diabetes was genetic. However, my grandparents were unaffected; the same with the aunts and uncles we were aware of along with my first cousins, *except* for a first cousin on my mother's side of the family, Barbara Jean. As told to me, this first maternal cousin was diagnosed with diabetes at the age of 24 or 25 somewhere in the late 1970's as I recall.

Before it became popular, I became acquainted with the possibility that stress, believe it or not, had something to do with the development of this disease in our family. I theorize that stress put upon my mother during her pregnancy with me may have been the cause, not neglecting the fact of my father's possible alcoholism.

Anguish is the best word I can use to describe my parents' feelings at the onslaught of this news. One of many stories my mother tells me is when she attempted to give me an insulin injection.

"Don't cry, mommy," from the mouth of this two-year old. "It will be okay."

And this became the first of many, *man*y, other shots until I learned how to do *it* myself.

Therefore, insulin introductions to our family became quickly absorbed as in being accepted; it became a necessity as water sustains life.

From my mother's recollections, my first type of insulin was called '*Lente*.' Known as an "intermediate-acting insulin, [it] covers insulin needs for about half the day or overnight. This type of insulin is often combined with rapid- or short- acting insulin." (**http://diabetes.webmd.com.**) For your convenience, an article link is pasted below listing the multiple types of insulins that are available today:

Type of Insulin & Brand Names	Onset	Peak	Duration	Role in Blood Glucose Management
Rapid-Acting				
Humalog or lispro	15-30 min.	30-90 min	3-5 hours	Rapid-acting insulin covers insulin needs for meals eaten at the same time as the injection. This type of insulin is used with longer-acting insulin.
Novolog or aspart	10-20 min.	40-50 min.	3-5 hours	
Apidra or glulisine	20-30 min.	30-90 min.	1-2½ hours	
Short-Acting				
Regular (R) humulin or novolin	30 min. -1 hour	2-5 hours	5-8 hours	Short-acting insulin covers insulin needs for meals eaten within 30-60 minutes
Velosulin (for use in the insulin pump)	30 min.-1 hour	2-3 hours	2-3 hours	
Intermediate-Acting				
NPH (N)	1-2 hours	4-12 hours	18-24 hours	Intermediate-acting insulin covers insulin needs for about half the day or overnight. This type of insulin is often combined with rapid- or short-acting insulin.
Lente (L)	1-2½ hours	3-10 hours	18-24 hours	
Long-Acting				
Ultralente (U)	30 min.-3 hours	10-20 hours	20-36 hours	Long-acting insulin covers insulin needs for about 1 full day. This

Lantus	1-1½ hour	No peak time; insulin is delivered at a steady level	20-24 hours	type of insulin is often combined, when needed, with rapid- or short-acting insulin.
Levemir or Detemir(FDA approved June 2005)	1-2 hours	6-8 hours	Up to 24 hours	
Pre-Mixed*				
Humulin 70/30	30 min.	2-4 hours	14-24 hours	These products are generally taken twice a day before mealtime.
Novolin 70/30	30 min.	2-12 hours	Up to 24 hours	
Novolog 70/30	10-20 min.	1-4 hours	Up to 24 hours	
Humulin 50/50	30 min.	2-5 hours	18-24 hours	
Humalog mix 75/25	15 min.	30 min.-2½ hours	16-20 hours	

*Premixed insulins are a combination of specific proportions of intermediate-acting and short-acting insulin in one bottle or insulin pen (the numbers following the brand name indicate the percentage of each type of insulin).

WebMD Medical Reference provided in collaboration with the Cleveland Clinic

The bolded insulin brand names are all of the types that I have ever used to date.

How does a doctor/physician choose which insulin would be the best for a patient, never mind a child patient? I honestly do not know. I think it is a hit or miss, experimental type of choice with the attitude of "Let's put you on this one;" or "Try this one and see if it works for you."

Going down the list, beginning with "Humalog," I was prescribed this brand in the mid-nineties. It made me physically and mentally ill. This was the ultimate reason that I purchased an insulin pump through the serious and frightening complication that I was literally going insane because of this disease. My personal experiences with the insulin pump are extravagantly explained in upcoming pages!

"Apidra" is my present insulin within the insulin pump. As I was told, it is *manufactured* with a buffer so as not to clog the infusion set tubing. Yes, I know; *manufactured* means *man-made*.

The "Regular" and "NPH" types were used by me, together, during my late teens to late thirties. It was quite an art to accomplishing the measuring and mixing of separate insulins in specific micrometer units to then inject in your own body. To this day, I have a sense of pride in being able to perform this so-called chore.

"Humalog" was a type of insulin that my sister, Gina, used. Yes, we are a family of multi-diabetics, also explained further on. She was allergic to it! At the time, I had never heard of a person being *allergic* to insulin. However, I have heard about such instances since her demise.

For personal reasons, I wanted to know the *ingredients* of the insulin I use. Inside each and every pre-packaged box of any and every insulin that I have ever been familiar with, are sheets of finely printed pages, usually two, that are not and never have been reader friendly – at least to me. Right at the beginning of one sheet it reads "Insulin aspart [DNA origin] Injection." What the heck is *that*? Not specific in its definition, once again I found my answer through simple internet research. It is partially quoted as follows with the website addresses that are provided for your interest and benefit if you choose:

"Insulin aspart-insulin aspart protamine, Generic Name: insulin aspart and insulin aspart protamine (IN su lin AS part, IN su lin AS part PRO ta meen).

"Brand names: *NovoLog Mix 70/30, NovoLog Mix 70/30 FlexPen, Novolog Mix 70/30 PenFill*

Official Site- LANTUS® (insulin glargine [rDNA origin] injection) Get Facts About LANTUS® www.LANTUS.com

Improve your blood sugar control.
Information and tips on insulin www.GoInsulin.com"

"What is insulin aspart and insulin aspart protamine?

"Insulin is a hormone that is produced in the body. It works by lowering levels of glucose (sugar) in the blood. Insulin aspart and insulin aspart protamine is a faster-acting form of insulin than regular human insulin. Insulin aspart and insulin aspart protamine is used to treat type 1 (insulin-dependent) diabetes in adults. Insulin aspart and insulin aspart protamine may also be used for other purposes not listed in this medication guide."

"What is the most important information I should know about insulin aspart and insulin aspart protamine?"

"Insulin aspart and insulin aspart protamine are fast-acting insulins that begin to work very quickly. After using it, you should eat a meal right away. Take care to keep your blood sugar from getting too low, causing hypoglycemia. Symptoms of <u>low blood sugar</u> (aka: hypoglycemia) may include, but are not limited to, a headache, feelings of nausea, hunger, confusion, drowsiness, weakness, dizziness, blurred vision, fast heartbeat, sweating, tremor, and/or trouble concentrating. Carry a piece of non-dietetic hard candy or glucose tablets with you in case you have low blood sugar. Also be sure your family and close friends know how to help you in an emergency.

"Also watch for signs of blood sugar that is too high (hyperglycemia). These symptoms include increased thirst, loss of appetite, increased urination, nausea, vomiting, drowsiness, dry skin, and dry mouth. Check your blood sugar levels and ask your doctor how to adjust your insulin doses if needed.

"Insulin aspart and insulin aspart protamine is only part of a complete program of treatment that may also include diet, exercise, weight control, foot care, eye care, dental care, and testing your blood sugar. Follow your diet, medication, and exercise routines very closely. Changing any of these factors can affect your blood sugar levels."

"What should I discuss with my healthcare provider before using insulin aspart and insulin aspart protamine?"

"Do not use this medication if you are allergic to insulin, or if you are having an episode of hypoglycemia (low blood sugar).

"Before using insulin aspart and insulin aspart protamine, tell your doctor if you have liver disease, kidney disease, or a nerve disorder.

"This medication is only part of a complete program of treatment that may also include diet, exercise, weight control, foot care, eye care, dental care, and testing your blood sugar. Follow your diet, medication, and exercise routines very closely. Changing any of these factors can affect your blood sugar levels.

"Your doctor will need to check your progress on a regular basis. Do not miss any scheduled appointments."

Although this description and definition does not answer my question, this is the best I could find through my personal research at this time. I have been under the impression that Novolog is man-made which leaves me feeling a bit quizzical due to my naturalness. Sure it works, and it works well. However just as pills are man-made, unnatural, long-term and unnatural effects are not expressed.

Returning the topic of my initial care when first diagnosed in 1959, I had to continue to use the "potty seat." In fact, I continued to have to use a variety of potty seats until I was 15 years old. Who knew? This was the easiest way to collect urine for absolute and necessary testing for glucose four times a day. However, due to school hours, it was done twice a day.

Using what is known as a "Clinitest kit" that was stored in the bathroom medicine cabinet; it smelled funny – horribly bad - and distinctive.

Five drops of urine with ten drops of water in a glass tube; drop in a tablet and watch it fizz, fizz, fizz as it turned colors: colors from bright blue, timid green, bright yellow or burning orange were displayed. Either of these colors indicated the level of glucose – sugar – in my bloodstream albeit through my urine. Yellow and orange gave the impression that the glucose level was high; whereas, green and blue were good, implying that the glucose level was low. The process was scary to see as a child and I certainly never ever wanted to touch one, afraid it would burn me.

Yes, quite odd, albeit historic, compared to the machination processes of today. In my mind, yellow and orange signified "bad" colors. This meant I did something wrong. Maybe I ate too much. Or maybe I ate something I wasn't supposed to eat. Those colors told me something was wrong with my body, my diabetes. Did I have an infection? Was my body giving me a signal for something? Fear. Fear introduced itself to me before I even knew what fear was.

For example, when Coco, our dog, bit my thumb while playing in the back yard with my older sister, my mother got so frightened. I was, perhaps, three years old.

"Infection, infection" she cried.

Her reaction and actions taken meant a severe scrubbing to get the germs out, you know, and then a dousing with merthiolate. Gosh that stung! Merthiolate and I became very well acquainted throughout my childhood. I don't know if it is sold any longer. But then again, I haven't looked for it either. Don't want to!

Gosh, the anxiety, the stress. Unbeknownst to the general public at the time, stress was not recognized in children; children didn't get "stressed out" supposedly. As a diabetic child, I have come to realize that stress does, in fact, offset my glucose readings, making them high. There is no other explanation. For example, the stress of a school bully, being bitten by my dog, or being scolded would upset my person, therefore my blood sugars. Sensitive, sensitive, sensitive.

And so, that was the last of Coco. I recall him/her being a blond or light brown colored dog, perhaps a golden Labrador Retriever or a Mastiff Pitbull of sorts. I just knew that daddy put him/her in his car, making Coco a vague memory for me. This incident was blamed for my fear of dogs that continued until long into my adulthood.

Ironically, as for the Clinitest testing procedure, the colors yellow and orange, are my favorite colors to this day. This type of testing, the only type available at the time in order to monitor glucose levels through urine, would continue for many years to come.

Chapter 2
"School days, school days…"

We moved again, to Newport, Rhode Island. My older sister and I became pupils of a private and former French-Catholic Elementary School, St. Cluny's in Newport, at the ages of six and four, respectively. Marcy, a delicate, boney, long-legged wisp of a girl with naturally yellow bologna curls that bounced as she walked, was always in a hurry; and I, heftier in stature, rounder in face, squared-shouldered, slower in gait, was always behind Marcy. I recall few things at that age. Those I do recall are quite poignant and in color, as in a dream.

An acceptable age to begin elementary school in that state at the time, Marcy and I were uniformed, combed, and brought to school every day by our mother, with our brown paper lunch bags in hand. I do not recall the present day collector's items of the metal lunch boxes. Those would come soon enough, oh yes.

One most prominent memory was the school play-ground and recess area. It was a vast, almost massive, expanse of green grass with a huge boulder at one side. Many, if not all the children, would race themselves silly to that rock at recess time. I recall having to get out of the way, staring at and watching the older children climb and push each other to get to the top of that rock.

Watching, viewing, seeing, and studying the importance of climbing that rock, I remained behind after the bell rang one afternoon, not returning to the typical line-up before re-entering the classroom. I had a mission and I accomplished it at the risk of being scolded by my teacher! I climbed that rock! But nobody was there. No one was there to root me on, to holler my name, to share in the witnessing of this conquering event! Oh well. I had to go in. In my scurry, I may have ripped my leotards or scratched a patent leather shoe that caused questions. I never told a soul, until now!

Another memory seems more of a vague and baffling instance as I share it with you now.

As was customary in that environment at the time, an afternoon nap was scheduled daily with the children, at least we kindergarteners. Lying upon my cot, "Sister" approached me with an apple in her hand. It was the apple from my lunch bag. It looked familiar. I may have seen mom pack it that morning along with my sister's lunch.

"Why did you bite this apple?" she asked. "I found it with your afternoon snack."

"I didn't want anyone else to eat it," I defensively replied. I recall that scene as the first of many to come in so, so, many attempts to take care of myself. Becoming defensive, assertive, and even aggressive developed and grew into me naturally, but was unrecognizable for many years to come.

Nonetheless, that particular instance was reported to my mother. This also became my first recollection of my eating requirements. Forever imbedded in my mind, the facts of when, where, why, how, and how much to eat began here. It also triggered a mental defense mechanism. Not only did I learn to defend my actions or inactions with this disease, I defended my mother, sisters, and even medical personnel for certain actions and inactions. This was a beginning to self-knowledge. I think of it now as rationalizing what, when, where, how, and how much I needed toward anything and everything. Perhaps an in-born trait, rationalizing, analyzing, albeit explaining my actions or inactions, especially when very young, was more to ease the ignorance of others. After all, this disease was not well-versed in 1960.

That was a monumental year in itself because Gina was born. "Eugenia Marie" was her Christian Baptismal name. This exciting and energetic little sister, child #4, was happy to see me after school. The earliest memory I have of her is clearly remembered. Walking in the front door of our house after school one day, Gina was bouncing and jumping and giggling and happy to see *me*! I dropped whatever I was holding, probably my school bag, and scurried over to where Gina was, in the play-pen. I scooched her up quickly and hugged her to me like she was a long lost puppy! That is a fond memory, a *very* fond memory.

The facts of a strict dietary regimen were shared with teachers throughout my early academic career which made all teaching personnel aware of this disease – *my* diabetes. I was a liability. If something were to happen to me, passing out, for instance, hell was going to be paid beginning through my mother! After all, and as far as I know to this day, I was the only juvenile diabetic throughout high school as well. That fact is astounding to me at this writing.

With diabetes being a *present day* epidemic and pandemic, newspaper and magazine articles are in abundance! Examples are displayed on page 23. Marketing ploys through television commercials portray many little children and their families, like me and mine, having been affected and effected with diabetes. There were certainly not as many other diabetics back then, back in 1960, as there are in existence today. Although I can appreciate a journalist's efforts to inform the public of any and all possible hope of defeat toward this unhealthy dilemma, I have become nonplussed.

Food "substitutions" or "exchanges" became very familiar as I grew older. Substitutions are a nice way of having and eating what you want. However, a sacrifice also has to be made. Consequences abound. For example, if I was offered an extra scoop of mashed potatoes, and accepted, I would need to forego my apple for dessert, staying within my daily caloric regimen. Or, a scoop of ice cream would cost me butter on my mashed potatoes, my milk, and my apple.

Overeating was not and is not an option. When in gluttonous moments, and I've had my share, believe me, I get sick. More insulin is required with some type of exercise exertion.

Food portions were measured and weighed for each and every meal until I was old enough to be familiar with portion sizes by sight. It is so-oo-o automatic for me now to look at all kinds of foods and knowingly measure an amount of insulin to react with each portion. A nasty trick was becoming familiar with sauces, gravies and the unseen ingredients that increased my blood sugar levels. Unless I became ill after a certain meal, I had to re-cap in my mind what I ate and then learned to increase my insulin and my exercise to break down those extra calories. Yes, food has been scary. To this day, eating out is a rare pleasure if only because I do not know what's in half the stuff I want to order and eat. And, no matter, my blood sugar skyrockets in every restaurant where I have eaten! So, I prefer to stay in my 'home element' and cook. Thank goodness I am a good cook!

As JoAnna M. Lund writes in *The Diabetic's Healthy Exchanges Cookbook*, "Exchange Lists are the heart and soul of the diabetic diet. Your doctor and/or dietitian will help you determine the [number of daily calories for your body type along with the] kind of exchanges you should use for your meals and snacks. So many variables, such as your age, your sex, how active you are, and whether you need to lose weight are considered when determining what is best for you. While the exchange lists are designed primarily for people with diabetes and others who must follow special diets, this information really just makes good nutrition sense."

I agree wholeheartedly. This extremely valuable information would/could wipe out the "obesity epidemic" of the 21st century.

The "special" with a diabetics' diet greatly involves timing, the scheduling of meals, and meal planning. Too many times I have been completely exasperated with family, extended family, friends, and their friends when it comes to dining out. My times are not *their* times; my choices of healthy eating places have not been *their* choice. Time and time again I play the role of martyr and sacrifice my well-being to make others happy. This mindset I blame on my Christian ethics. There just came a time in my life that I finally asserted myself to just say "no" or try to explain to people, once again, that I am diabetic and need this and so forth.

Such instances have tried my patience, leaving me to feel embarrassed and humiliated because *they* refuse to respect my requests without a long explanation of "why." I've lost people in my life because I found them to be just plain disrespectful, thoughtless, to my living requirements. You know the saying "you can count your friends on one hand." Well, this is very true for me. This includes helpful people, concerned people, understanding and appreciative people. These choice few I've known for decades now.

Re-locating as a family from Newport, Rhode Island, to Worcester, Massachusetts, in 1963, with four children and one on the way, my parents, especially my mom, were excited about owning their first home. Uncle John, one of my mother's older brothers, helped build it for her, his career being a home building contractor/construction worker.

Known as a "California Ranch House," our new home was built purposely with three bedrooms, one bath, and a full basement. Uncle John made sure that the placement of all light switches, the design and placement of the bathroom sink and bathtub, the low shelving in the closets, and the safety factors and ease of use for his nieces and nephew were complete. For instance, light switches in every room were lower than normal for a child to be able to reach. The same "lower" design accompanied the shelving in all the closets. They were low enough for a child to reach the items that were stored.

The cellar ended up being the most fun place for me at times. Through a door in the upstairs hall and 14 steps down, Marcy and I slowly navigated our way down. Exploring the area, we realized that this space duplicated the upstairs spacing without details. There were two inner walls, one of which held the stairs. There was a door to the backyard, and three windows, one on the north side, one on the south side, and one in the middle, facing east. The east window, on the same side as the door, was the only one Marcy and I could open. The others were too high. The rest of the cellar was wide open, making it possible for Marcy and I to ride our bikes, play house, play school, or play 'tag, you're it'. Playing tag was the best game.

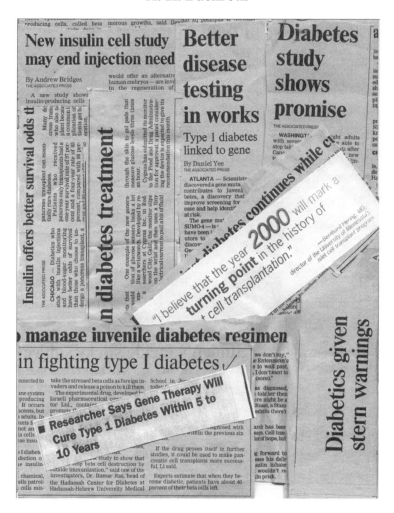

Soon enough, dad painted the concrete cellar floor and walls 'navy grey.' So very appropriate for a Navy man. "Why everything that color, dad," I asked. "Because it's free. I took it off the ship" he replied. I understood. After all the walls and floor had dried, dad took a third of that cellar space for his tool shop with a separate doorway entrance. The hot water heater was inside that space too. Mom used the way-back-area for storing winter coats, boots, ice skates, trunks, seasonal decorations, and other haunting cellar belongings. Shelves were built, drawers put in, closets formed, and the rest was ours. Our board games were stacked down there in a special spot and matured as we all did ("Candyland," "Mouse Trap,"

"The Game of Life," "Scrabble," "Chinese Checkers," etc.). The Barbie Dolls also had their own spot with all their attachments: wardrobes, boyfriends (including G. I. Joe), accoutrements and accessories. What we didn't have for the Barbies, we made – a cardboard car or a living space.

As an older sister, I was able and expected to help settle with the little ones; putting things away; remembering where other things were. There were lots of little responsibilities for Marcy and me as we were "big girls" now. We had designated responsibilities that we took seriously.

It was a busy summer: meeting the neighborhood kids; meeting aunts, uncles and cousins that already lived there; starting a vegetable garden with dad; capturing butterflies; getting manure from a cow farm for the garden; picking out rocks for the back yard patio. I remember this stuff.

Part of this adjustment included an immediate enrollment for all of us with the areas' government medical facilities. However, medicinal supplies for me were concentrated upon furthering my life, not necessarily enhancing it. My siblings were unclaimed by diabetes – at this time. Insulin was the trick. One shot every morning of every day to assist in the digestion of food. My little pancreas did not work. Because of this fact, I could not eat lollipops, tootsie rolls, birthday cakes, etc. There is sugar in that stuff, yucky, icky, bad sugar that would make me literally sick. I may as well have been allergic to sugar and any food item that contained it! Therefore, it was drilled into my head by repetitions that any form of sugar was off limits EXCEPT when necessary to alleviate a hypoglycemic reaction (aka: "reaction" or "insulin reaction," meaning there is too much insulin in the body with nothing for it to work on/digest). Sharing with school mates' birthday parties was absolutely forbidden! I always felt that their parents were afraid of me with this disease. I learned alienation.

Taking a shot every day was common to me, personally, and my immediate family. But my little school and neighborhood friends had no idea. Therefore, my secret continued.

My siblings also had a secret, the same secret. Too many times my older sister had to sacrifice social events due to watching over me. This continued well into adolescence. It was useless to say "I can't go because my sister has diabetes and I have to watch her." It was just easier for her to say "I have to babysit." Nobody knew what the disease was except those that had it and their medical personnel. Older folks referred to it as "having sugar." I didn't and do not "have sugar." I have diabetes. That never made much sense to me.

Eminent with this re-location, we had to transfer to a new school. Due to the different states' age enrollment laws, specifically being between Rhode Island and Massachusetts at the time, Marcy was able to enter second grade with no problem. I entered kindergarten with no problem, however, I was withheld a year because I was too young.

At the end of that particular school year, I watched all my classmates proceed through the school's corridors to first grade. Sister Marilyn, the kindergarten teacher, physically held me. I wanted to go with them, upstairs, to where all the bigger kids were. I wanted to be with my friend, Linda. Wasn't I big enough? Why couldn't I go? I was confused, sad. I didn't understand. No one explained. I stayed behind with Sister Marilyn not knowing why as she and I awaited the arrival of new pupils.

After the initial hubbub, life proceeded on as normal. At the end of the day and once arriving home, my mother explained the circumstances to me. I accepted it and moved on. I liked school. I made new friends and acquaintances, excelling in the kindergarten learning process because I had done this all already. I became Sister Marilyn's helper, knowing where the class supplies – crayons, paper, scissors, song books, etc. - were kept. This experience taught me responsibility if not for myself, for others as well. It was like being a big sister in a bigger environment. Heck, I knew how to get around: through the big doors, outside to the sidewalk, down the hill through the parking lot to the side-door of the Church, down the stairs to the Church basement for lunch, and back again, safely, showing the new kids how to do the same. If we weren't accompanied by Sister Marilyn, then a high school girl would volunteer. The high school girls were always more fun because they were real people, although in uniform. Be that as it may, I remember sharing with Sister Marilyn that I wanted to be a nun when I grew up. She was delighted, of course, telling my mother who thought that idea was absolutely glorious. I was deemed to be a "good girl."

After enrollment in St. Mary's Elementary School, we, as a family, also became parishioners of Our Lady of Chęstochowa Catholic Church. The historical background of this Church and school deals predominantly with Poland. As a family of six, there was a time when we attended a Sunday morning Mass there together. This parish was the community's and the area's only Polish Catholic Church. A typical, early morning Sunday Mass constituted detailed preparations the night before to include, but not limit, the pressing and setting out of dresses, hats, gloves and mantillas along with the polishing of patent leather shoes with Vaseline. My mother wanted to make a better than good impression. She and her family belonged to this parish. She grew up in this ethnic city and its Polish neighborhood known as "Vernon Hill." She went to elementary school at St. Mary's. There was an automatic presumption that most of the city's Polish people lived around here, in this neighborhood. Not only was the Polish school and Church available, but the specialty markets for Polish appetites. Ah yes, Polish appetites with their kielbasas, bulka rolls, babka (cakes), and tortes. Italians lived a few miles away on Shrewsbury Street; the Irish lived on and around "Green Street" with a mix on Vernon Street. My mother's re-establishing her family here marked the beginning of my Polish pupilage. This was extremely important to my mother although her children were born of mixed ethnicity.

Recalling my first visit to our Lady of Częstochowa, I accompanied my parents and siblings. Walking down that ever-so-long Church aisle for the first time with my dad on one side, cradling a wriggling baby brother, Charles, with Marcy and mom on my right side, while mom held our baby sister, Gina, we proceeded through the huge front doors and down the ever-so-long Church aisle. As we approached a pew toward the front of the Church, near the altar, I became absolutely awestruck at the beauty. I recall this vividly. The colorful paintings depicting biblical scenes along with the overwhelming brightness of the gorgeous stained-glass windows left me breathless. The majestic, multi-colored details of the sainted characters with their symbols of animals or vases or baskets beholding detailed depictions of varying fruits, flowers or grasses popped out at me. I could almost touch the colors. There are too many times to count how many times I walked that aisle.

Not only did those multi-colored, stained glass windows seem 10' tall, but the portraiture of paintings over the altar and sacristy with life-size depictions of Jesus Christ and his disciples remain breathtaking. No, I did not know who or what these paintings represented at the time. That knowledge would all fall into place through my pupilage at St. Mary's Elementary School.

Nonetheless, that day I began speaking with the main character in the center of this painting, Jesus Christ himself! I remember having been frightened at this larger-than-life persona yet concerned with wonderment at what it all meant. Illusions ran away with me at each and every visit to that Church thereafter. Heck, I wasn't quite six years old.

I don't specifically recall what we discussed, Jesus and I. It seemed that Jesus always had something to tell me. I distinctly remember Him nodding His head to me at times, looking at me – only me - during my visits.

Many, many times I found mental and emotional relief in that Church under the eyes of Jesus. I shared concerns about being sick, worries about my parents, worries about my siblings and whatever else my young world experienced.

Such conversations continued until deep into junior high. No one knew. Another secret. As a child, this divine influence inflamed a spiritual vision that I was going to be all right. This was between the Christ Child and me, but it spread to my seeing angels. On three separate occasions in my mothers' home, visions of these beloved, holy entities appeared. For instance, there was a time when I was chastised and sent to bed early. Awakened in darkness, the Blessed Mother Mary appeared to me, flanked with an angel on each side of her. Her garb was a light blue gown with a white veil, as pictured in my religion book. The angels stood silently beside her, all white with their wings folded back. Her words to me were "You will be all right." Speechless and in awe, I fell back to sleep, exclaiming this vision to my mother the next morning.

An enlightening book entitled *Ask Your Guides* by Sonia Choquette, reads in part that "…children have a far greater chance of consciously connecting and interacting with their angels than adults do because their hearts are so open and their spirits are so strong. In fact, kids are even taught angel-invoking prayers, but adults believe themselves to be too sophisticated for such intimacies."

Angel of God, guardian dear,
To whom God's love commits me here,
Ever this day, be at my side
To light, to guard, to rule and guide.

I could probably have been labeled "delusional." I don't care. I saw what I saw and on more than one occasion. Jesus and I spoke to each other through our minds, developing my ever-present soul, intuition, a strong faith, and beliefs. Awesome. He became and remains my strength. Angels, as messengers of God, remain at my side. I believe.

Back in those days, the early '60's, nuns were garbed in black, floor-length attire called "habits" with a medieval type black cloth veil that cascaded over their shoulders. A white cloth piping was atop this head-piece similar to a head-band to hold the veil in place. Nuns had no hair, at least not that I could see. In my child's mind, nuns were not people. I mean, they were not human. And they had no feet that I could see because of the length of their habits. Rather frightening if you think about it! Their gowns swept the halls and the stairs, and were quite overwhelming when seen swooshing about in an emergency or a tempest of some sort or another. As time went on, perhaps the 1970's, trends did as well. Their skirts became shorter, the veils shortened as well, allowing nuns to show hair. I could actually see the nuns' shoes acknowledging to me that they really did have feet!

Within the Polish alphabet, the "W" is pronounced as an English "V" and the crossed "L" is pronounced as a "W." Yes, I was in school with names such as "Burszynska," "Mikolajczyk," "Lewandowski," "Oslowski," "Mrugała," "Rudzinska," "Kusz," "Swierzbien," "Slowatyczki", "Jeznach," "Chesna," "Gustowska," "Gawronska," "Jachimczyk," "Lemanski," "Milewska," "Zielonka," "Prizio,"and more! Then there were us, the "Buckroths," along with the "Dymeks," a "Matys," a "Morrissey," a "Stanick," the "Meehans," the "Kuberts" and "McNallys," the "Lawrences," and a "Mahoney."

Occasionally, a few Polish children/classmates could not speak English when arriving at our school. While as children, my English speaking classmates and I helped to teach them English and in return we learned Polish with a large exchange of laughter. Pronouncing the Polish names as a child enhanced my Polish speaking and writing skills to this day. Please excuse me if any of these recognized names are misspelled.

The teachers were all nuns except for one, Miss Joanne, the sixth grade mathematics teacher. The introduction of 'lay teachers' expanded as the grades progressed and times changed. As a group, the nuns were known as "Sisters of the Holy Family of Nazareth." They had names such as: Sr. Marilyn (Kindergarten); Sr. Elaine (first grade); Sr. Cyrene (second grade); Sr. Consilia (third grade); Sr. Remigina (fourth grade); Miss Patricia (fifth grade); Sr. Joanita (sixth grade); Miss Natalie (seventh grade); and Sr. Anne (eighth grade). The onslaught of high school introduced us to Srs. Eleanor (Spanish), Cathleen (Biology), and Peter (English); Miss Helen Lewinska (Latin); and Mr. Palazzi (History). Once again, please excuse the name spellings and even the grade progression of each teacher. I would like to give the memory of Sister Remigina credit for my love of history, spelling, and vocabulary (synonyms, homonyms, acronyms, etc.). To me, she was a kindly, grandmotherly-type woman with sparkling, kind blue eyes and a constant calming expression. Her physical stature was that of a teddy-bear: short, round and plump. She seemed huggable, but I never hugged her. Implied protocol. I often saw compassion in her eyes, as if she felt sorry for me for being a diabetic. I could just tell, not prove. I would like to give the memory of Sister Anne credit for my fondness of writing, correctly, the English language. She also taught me the proper way of sweeping a floor, using a broom and dustpan. As this was my main and daily chore at home, I was thankful to be able to learn how to do this task properly without swooshing dust around.

There was a very special occasion at the school one year when former Boston Red Sox baseball player, Carl Yastrzemski, visited our school. Not only a 'Pole,' but he was a famous baseball player that lived in our home state and played for our home town team. That was quite encouraging for all of us little Polish kids especially those with such tremendous Polish sir names. Learning the Polish language was not only a requirement at that school beginning in first grade, but one talent I wish I was more practiced in at present. I repeatedly attempt to keep up with that language, which is good exercise for my brain.

One special friend I made in this second semester of kindergarten is Ricky Wołosz. Ricky and I remain acquainted to this day, although distant. We sat next to each other in most classes and always tried to continue to sit next to each other throughout our school days. High school was a different story. We graduated high school together as with so many of the other kindergarteners at the time. You see, St. Mary's not only supplied a Polish Catholic Church, but an elementary school with attached high school as well. My attendance continued through those halls for 13 years until graduation with 41 kids in my graduation class. From thereon in, I was always astounded at public school graduations having an excess of 300+ high school graduates.

A recollection of Ricky's attentions to my diabetes happened when Marcy came into our kindergarten classroom one day, totally exacerbated, anxious, as I recall. She strongly told Ricky and whomever was sitting with us at the kindergarten table that "she (meaning me) didn't eat candy because it would make her sick and don't let her eat any candy." Her concern was flattering to me but disconcerting to Ricky. Any other child within earshot certainly didn't know what she meant, or why, in her hurried flurry. As the oldest of five children, she was probably prompted by mom to talk to my friends. She was learning to protect me. Her protection was often embarrassing, as she 'policed' me at times.

From there on in, Ricky became my guardian of sorts, a true friend. Now *he* had a responsibility without knowing it! Marcy, I'm sure, must have felt a bit relieved to be able to shed some of the responsibility of having to take care of her little sister. Gosh, being the oldest of five children was gruesome enough!

Because of that incident, it was plain to see that all the kids knew that I couldn't eat lollipops, tootsie rolls, birthday cakes, the ever-popular blonde cake-with-cream, *Twinkies*; the chocolate cake and cream tubules covered in chocolate called *Ho-Ho's*; the 2-in-a-pack chocolate covered *Ding-Dongs*, etc. Ah, that killed me. My mouth watered just looking at those edible temptations!

All these goodies, and more, were available at the little store at the top of the hill from school. The location of that store was an *excellent* marketing idea and physical position. It appealed to the children with money, the supposedly more financially well-off kids that went to this private school down the street. More convenient was the ever-popular bus stop, right there. While so many of us waited after school for the City bus downtown to transfer to another one, or the bus that took me and mine straight home, there was time to linger in that little store. Sure, I went in. I lingered. I longed. But I did not buy anything. The specific quarter in my pocket was for the bus ride. The dime in my pocket was "in case of emergency," to telephone mom at work if I needed to. That dime got pretty old because it stayed in my pocket for a very long time.

Sure, I have had all of the above-mentioned treats sooner or later, in secret, somewhere. Because I was not supposed to eat this stuff, and everybody around me knew I was not supposed to eat this stuff, temptation and curiosity got the best of me. As I got older and my allowance increased, I started to cheat. That is, I cheated on my stringent diet. The consumption of any sugared confection required that I crouch behind a stairwell, or behind a closed restroom stall door, or behind a locker door. Once knowing I was out of view of any one's eyes, I would stuff all of whatever it was into my mouth. Gobbling in such a fashion, I didn't even taste it. That acknowledgement gave me reason to try another one, at another time, when I could eat it more slowly and enjoy it – *savor it* - whatever *it* happened to be! Not only was I a "cheat," but I slowly became a "sneak."

Going to school mates' birthday parties was absolutely forbidden! Remember, I adamantly feel that their parents were afraid of me with this disease. They didn't understand, nor appreciate the challenges of this disease. *It* was uncommon and certainly not popular. I remained alienated.

I did have an opportunity to share in a best friend's 8th birthday. It's the only birthday celebration that I recall being able to attend. Her name was Pamela and her mom was a registered nurse. That fact alone allowed my mother to let me attend. Pamela's mother made this event more special for the both of us by taking Pam and I to a nearby supermarket so I could pick out 'something special,' something just for me to eat, something I felt comfortable with. I chose a stock of celery. Yep, a simple stock of celery. I knew that I could eat all of that if I wanted and not get sick in any way shape or form. Not only was celery safe for me, but other people around me were safe in knowing that I would be safe and happy. Oh yes, I became ever so aware of making the correct choices if not only for myself, but for others' peace of mind. I'll never forget that party. It was redeeming for my soul, a mature and happy experience for my friend and her family. To this day, I greatly enjoy eating celery and have learned that not only is it a great source of fiber for cleaning out my colon, but also has "the power to help neutralize uric acid and other excess acids in the body." (*Bottom Line's Healing Remedies* by Joan Wilen and Lydia Wilen.)

During this time period, my parents separated. Dad left. My siblings and I learned to survive and take care of each other as best as we could through my mother's insistence, persistence, and discipline. It wasn't easy. And it took a long time. It took a long time to actually realize that he was not coming back; that he was not allowed back into our lives. Heartbreak city!

It became a defense in my mind, a creation, to dissuade others from knowing me, knowing my label, knowing I am diabetic with the further dramatization of being an abandoned, fatherless child. A normal, albeit non-diabetic life without having been ostracized, being cast out, being unacceptable, and non-invite-able to too many functions became an intangible "unwanted" sign on facial expressions and within unexpressed words. It's a sensing, really, a reaction to and noticing of body language. Such unkind *inactions* hurt and people don't know. Imagine, year after year, your classmates inviting other classmates, boys and girls, to their birthday parties but you're not invited, ever. My overhearing their party plans - who would be there, what present to bring, and what was to be eaten - made me feel bad because I was not invited. Nobody wanted me there.

My parents' separation added to this anxiety, to being ostracized. Such a thing, especially in a Catholic home with five children in the 1960's did not happen. This caused my mother to be 'excommunicated' from the Church. The fact of the matter might as well have been posted in the Church's' weekly newsletter, for heaven's sake! No matter how quiet I and my siblings were about *this* matter, everyone knew anyway.

We evidently and silently became utterly alone with each other.

My Diabetic Soul

It has occurred to me that life, among many descriptions, is an insurmountable excursion for many people. Those that take advantage of their health, their total well-being, their undiagnosed state-at-present will, eventually, be diagnosed with *something*. Sound too doomsayer-ish? No matter. It's fate. Everybody has *something* wrong with their body. I am convinced. A human body becomes worse when disrespected by its owner.

Before supper one school-day evening, Marcy and I were discussing what our souls could look like. After all, being enrolled in a private Catholic school, our religion classes inspired such a thought. Especially in preparation for the ever-important "First Holy Communion" at that age, this celebration is equated with great respect. We were approximately 8 and 6 years old, respectively.

What does any soul look like?

"Mine looks like a sword with a snake wrapped around it" I remember saying.

"Mine looks like a black box," Marcy said. "It's a square." She drew it in the air over the kitchen table.

Hmm. Not realizing at the time the full thrust of these thoughts, I now know that the visual of my soul came from the medical prescriptions that my life depended upon. This medical insignia was a constant subliminal message. No wonder. Through internet research, I found the meaning of this symbol and share it with you below. Yes, it is the cover of this book.

> *"The **caduceus** is the legendary herald's wand of the Greek God Hermes (Roman, Mercury). This symbol, a winged staff entwined by twin serpents, is nearly universal, found in Egypt, Mesopotamia, and India, where it is always a symbol of harmony and balance. The symbol may have originally been a symbol of the sovereignty of the Goddess Tanit.*
>
> *"It has been mistakenly utilized as a symbol of the medical industry in the place of the wand of Asclepius (Asculapius).*

"In the Hermetic Tradition, the caduceus is a symbol of spiritual awakening, and has been likened to the Kundalini serpents of Hindu mysticism."

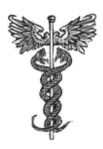

However, in one of my copies of The Holy Bible Revised Standard Version © 1952, is found a story involving the Canaanites with the king of Arad, fighting against the Israelites, this symbol was initialized by the Lord God Himself!

"From Mount Hor they set out by the way to the Red Sea, to go around the land of Edom; and the people became impatient on the way. And the people spoke against God and against Moses, "Why have you brought us up out of Egypt to die in the wilderness? For there is no food and no water, and we loathe this worthless food.

"Then the Lord sent fiery serpents among the people, and they bit the people, so that many people of Israel fled. And the people came to Moses, and said, "We have sinned, for we have spoken against the Lord and against you; pray to the lord, that He take away the serpents from us.

"So Moses prayed for the people.

And the Lord said to Moses, "Make a poisonous serpent, and set it on a pole; and everyone who is bitten shall look at it and live. So Moses made a serpent of bronze and put it upon a pole; and whenever a serpent bit someone, that person would look at the serpent of bronze and live."
~ Numbers 21:4-9 ~

As far as Marcy's description, that is her explanation, her concept, her vision, her story. Marcy, an extremely thin child with a characterization of self-determination mixed with stubbornness, had become an adult at the age of eight. A beautifully tall, long-legged child with long, curly blond hair, she dreamed of being a ballerina. Although that dream did not come to fruition, responsibilities overtook her life as the eldest child of five in a fatherless home in 1964. She is my "big sister." I looked up to her. We never were friends, Marcy and I. Although we are 2+ years apart biologically and went to the same schools, shared the same bed and bedroom, clothes, siblings, chores and responsibilities, we were never friends. That realization is sorrowful to me. My diabetes took too much attention.

Elementary school days - oh, precious childhood! – began with a urine test; then a shot that was often accompanied by bleeding and a small bruise – no big deal because it was so commonplace; then a balanced breakfast of oatmeal or cream of wheat, a hardboiled egg or a slice of cheese, a small glass of orange juice and a small glass of milk used for the oatmeal, sprinkled with salt. My brother and sisters had the same. Summer cereal breakfasts were replaced by Cheerios or Rice Krispies. You would never find sugar-coated cereals in our house. No, no, no!

I was always hungry. Not learning until well into my twenties that insulin makes you hungry, it makes sense to me now to know *why* I was always looking for someone to share his or her school lunch with me. Knowing that that was forbidden, I didn't care. I was hungry!

For example, I remember a moment when the school bell rang after lunch. Not allowed to eat during classes, a child had spat out a "hot ball" candy as we all gathered to line up and return to class. Rolling toward my feet, I picked it up, wiped it off, threw it in my mouth, and chewed, hurriedly, with glee. Silly? No, this was an opportunity! I certainly didn't want to face a reprimand from my teacher for eating something that I wasn't supposed to! Never mind that it was dirty from rolling down the hard top. Yes, teachers were informed of my being diabetic. Remember, I was the only one throughout grammar and high school that I ever knew of that was a diabetic. And I remained at St. Mary's for 13 years, until high school graduation. Alone. Secrets were kept back then, back in the late '60's. And not just about "having a deadly disease," if you know what I mean!

Lunch time in the cafeteria, located in the basement of the church, consisted of the bagged lunch that mom packed the night before. This was a time, part of an era, when small cartons of milk were 4¢ and there was no "hot lunch" program. All the kids "brown-bagged" it, and this was a chore done every night before bed in order to be ready to leave the house for school in the morning. At least that's how it was done in our house. However, there were too many times at school that there wasn't enough milk to go around causing me and some others to go without those sustaining calories.

Being on a stringent diet, this usually caused me to have an "insulin reaction" in the afternoon. I would pass out at my desk only to regain consciousness in the nurses' room, ingesting envelopes of white sugar, those usually kept and used for coffee drinkers. That's what was available. After 20 minutes, I was sent back to my class to resume whatever it was that was going on. No questions were asked. The other kids just knew "that Andrea got sick again." That was part of my reputation – "getting sick in school." Many of those low blood sugar reactions would start up again on the bus ride home from school. Unbeknownst to me or school authorities at the time, I should have had something more beneficial to eat within 20 minutes of eating the sugar.

To make matters worse, I didn't recognize the usual signs of hypoglycemia: the sweating, the shaking, and my inability to speak. I could feel them, but didn't realize that they were "a sign" of a low blood sugar reaction. The symptoms came on so fast; I could not grasp their meaning or the consequential intents. I could think and recall what happened, as it happened, but I couldn't use my tongue or my voice to speak. If and when I did, my words were garbled, incoherent. No one could understand what I was saying. However, in my head, I knew what I was saying and tearfully blurted it out once composure was regained. Being "non-symptomatic" as I phrase it, lasted until I was at least 11 years old. Could this inaction have been denial at such a young age? I don't know. I do know now that those 'signs' were my initiation to "reactions" as well as the enlightenment that I had to take care of myself! Occasionally, I "received a signal" where my eyes would cross. It didn't happen all the time. But I did recognize this after a few instances and knew that I was going to need juice. Making this proclamation to my mother, she was ecstatic that I was finally able to recognize a hypoglycemic reaction.

As briefly mentioned above, there were many such episodes after school hours. Walking up the steep hill from school to get to the bus stop, waiting for the bus, and walking the length of our street to the house was exerting and tiresome for me. Often times I could have fallen down in the street and fallen asleep. I felt weakness. But I always pushed on, forward into the house, leading the way for my younger siblings. I didn't want them to have to worry about me. There was too much going on in our little lives as it was. This was *my* secret.

I hung on until dinner. In an automaton state, I completed my chores, many times not thoroughly. This lack of thoroughness often resulted in a punishment or a chastisement of some sort. My older sister and I would prepare supper each day, awaiting mom's arrival home. Marcy was often critical of me saying "What's the matter with you? Why did you do that? Answer me! Can't you talk?!" As she pushed me out of the way, I didn't talk. She became angry, unintentionally, but it was there. She could not read my body signs never mind my mind. You see, not only are there body language signs that designate trouble (e.g., sweating, shaking, eyes rolling, speechlessness, body jerks, etc.), there is a certain developed lingo that goes along with this disease as well. For example, words and phrases such as "reaction," "gluco," "food," "juice," "pump up the jam," or "jam" are familiar to either another diabetic or a very familiar someone, such as a friend or relative when I am in their company.

Becoming aware – and being aware – of my body and all its functions has been vitally important!

When reporting such instances to my mother, I couldn't explain my actions or inactions. I was dubbed "dimwitted." Marcy seemed to delight in this. Already nicknamed "skinny-minny," I unconditionally joined this - whatever it was – club of name-calling. At least Marcy wasn't alone.

Needless to say, the "before supper clinitest testing" displayed the glorious "blue" on these days. In my mind, I celebrated, alone. The suffering was worth it, the sacrifice was worth it, if only to have an "acceptable" urine test reading. It was always a relief to me to see that color in the test tube. After all, as Catholics we were taught to suffer in order to gain glory in the eyes of God. "Suffer the little children…"

I didn't and don't consciously choose to sacrifice, per se. I just want to live and experience everything I can. This disease has egged me on to accomplish, adventure, experience, all things before I die.

With all my mind-boggling physical attention that needed heeding, more dramatic changes were to be burned into my childhood memories. As mentioned, not only were our parents "separated", but my maternal grandmother passed away; I went to summer camp and learned how to give my own insulin injections; plastic syringes became available; and another sister, Judy, was born. All this within a years' time!

Sister Elaine, our first grade teacher, was an eloquent, young, pretty, and kindly woman. I happened to cause her to freak out one class day as I volunteered to get some class supplies from a nearby hall cabinet. The white aluminum cabinet door was always stuck, making it hard to open. After fidgeting with it, I balanced my left arm on one corner and pulled using all my strength with my right hand. Well, didn't the corner of that cabinet door skid across the inside of my left arm, leaving a bloody gash? I ran back in the class room, holding my wounded arm. Sister Elaine gasped with horror, leading me to the nurses' station. The word "infection" was mentioned.

Returning to class, to Sr. Elaine, my arm bandaged of course, I was exhausted. It was an emotional exhaustion that I didn't immediately recognize. This led to a low blood sugar reaction. Good timing with our lunch and recess, the right time of day. Another one of those little blessings. I felt better after eating, as always. To this day I *always* feel better after I eat, even when I cannot decide whether I am hungry or not! Silly.

That specific cabinet disappeared the next day, never to be seen again.

I can only imagine the impression, or the memories, I left for my classmates. Perhaps I'll never know. This further proves to me how this disease has affected so many other people, especially with its present-day popularity, so to speak. I'm sure my name has been reiterated time and time again in conversations with "I once knew a girl that was a diabetic…"

I think that many of my grade school chums remember me to this day as being "sick." There were too many things that I could not eat, too many things that I could not do. People were afraid of me. I have always had the impression that they thought I was not going to make it too far in life.

Our mandatory school uniforms were not only considered respectable, neat and clean, but they were cost efficient as well. Girls' uniforms consisted of a navy blue wool-and-poly-mix jumper with a white, short-sleeved, button-down blouse with a 'Peter Pan' collar. A required bright red cross-bow-tie snapped at the throat. White ankle socks or knee socks were worn with black and white oxford shoes with laces. Boys had to wear dark-colored dress pants (preferably black or navy blue colored) with formal long or short-sleeve button down shirts with button cuffs and black ties. Socks matching the pants, of course, with leather topped black shoes were the norm. If parents could afford the blazers (woolen suit jackets for both sexes), then those were available. There weren't many blazers from my recollections.

The white knee socks I wore are what I need to stress. You see, feet care for a diabetic is especially essential. With that in mind, I was brought up to believe that the wearing of white socks would aid in the prevention of a foot infection. This implied suggestion told me that there was something about the dye in colored socks that could exacerbate a possible infection. This belief stayed with me all the way through high school, with my sister's hand-me-down socks, the elastic stretched, and the heels worn out, the socks continuously falling to my ankles. Wearing hand-me-down socks was embarrassing, but I did not have a choice at the time. Not until high school through having an after school job was I able to afford panty-hose, my favorites being the dark shaded "opaques." I still favor wearing these types of stockings. Even though they were colored - navy blue, black, gray and white were acceptable with the uniform - I needed to be stylin'. Remember, as all teenagers, I was invincible as well. Nothing was going to happen to me. It's the other guy or gal. All in all, there were no resultant or emergent catastrophes from wearing the colored panty hose.

Massachusetts snow and I became quite acquainted. It happened every winter of course. You know that. It didn't take us children long to expect it, look forward to it. With the chilly start of autumns' September school days, part of the "back-to-school" purchase included such gear as rubber boots, ugly galoshes (aka: "rubbers," which were literally protective rubber shoe covers in one color - brown), woolen hats, gloves, jackets if one of us or the other needed one item or the other. Hand-me-downs were consistent yet boring and quite unfashionable. Tolerable but unfashionable.

In my childish eyes, snow was always a majestic, sparkling clean blanket that covered the world, my world. This consisted of our immediate back yard and neighborhood. The "swamp" behind our house - a natural animal and plant sanctuary made up of four acres of wet land - was a fantastic sight to awaken to after a snow fall. Better still with a heavy snow fall was the cancellation of school.

With that in mind, the five of us were out the door right after breakfast. Tumbling over each other down the cellar stairs, we couldn't move fast enough to find and dig out our warm and heavy winter gear. Helping each other bundle up, per moms' supervision, we couldn't move too freely. Tucked and tied, we usually began our snow excursion by tramping out the cellar door and up the hill to the front yard with a shared sled in tow.

Sleds, being an absolute necessity in Massachusetts and probably most of New England, were wooden with metal brackets and sliders for easy play, easy sliding, dragging and pulling in the snow and ice. That's its purpose! Ours was a light colored wood with red stripes and red sliders. The colors, however, along with most of the varnish wore off due to constant use. This one sled with three to four children took quite a beating, as we took turns using it. We were taught as a group that such a toy had to be taken care of: wiped dry before being put back in the cellar and an occasional waxing of the sliders with a candle helped to make it slide even faster!

An excited hurry to make our way to the snow covered front-yard-hill was energy in motion! Cumbersome under layers of bulky clothes, the weight of the snow caused each of us, in turn, to collapse in roars of laughter only to get up again and trod up that hill! Determination in motion! Once there, we older girls voted that we slide down the hill first to making a path through the yard. Sure, the exertion was tiring just trying to plow through. Once accomplished, we zoomed down the hill, taking a younger sibling with us as only two could fit on the sled at one time. After years of such repeated play, the exertion was habitual and welcomed. Sheer fun! Eventually, mom promotes us to a toboggan wherein three of us could fit on that at one time.

"Andrea, come get your snack" mom would holler from a window or the back door. I could never tell where her voice came from. But she was there, watching us from inside the house. "Okay" I yelled back in a big voice, discerning that the time of day was 10:00am. This became a mental calculation toward how much time was left before lunch at noon and how much longer we could all stay out and play. Time certainly went by quickly and we still had snow and ice patches to conquer with snow men and women to build! Once getting the usual 10:00 Graham Crackers, I was ready to keep going. Exercise, exercise, and more exercise!

Tiring of the sled, we were off to the morass of swamp, located behind and adjacent to my mother's property. In actuality, these four acres of open land are an animal refuge. Flocks of all types of birds could often be seen from the bedroom windows. I especially enjoyed watching pheasants enter our yard and pick at the grass for worms. Frogs were abundant with their "ribbeting" sounds echoing the neighborhood night and day through the spring and summer while our adventures of catching them led to streams and streams of pollywogs. Wild rabbits were numerous as rabbits are known to be, along with snakes and creatures of deep and hidden hiding places.

My sisters, brother and I frequented this area throughout the years. Under a blanket of snow, these creatures of nature slept. We knew we wouldn't disturb a living thing as we climbed over large clumps of weedy grass and uprooted reeds. One such investigative adventure brought us to a small iced water hole. The way we discovered this delight was by slipping and sliding all over it and each other. Brushing away the cover of heavy, thick snow with our hands, feet, and legs, we determined that it was solid ice. Delighted, we just had to get back to the cellar, find our ice skates, dust them off and put them on! In high expectations, we were not permitted to continue this adventure until after lunch.

With that being done in a harmonious rush, we regained our energies and re-clothed ourselves and each other whether our clothes were wet or not. We *had* to get out there! All ice skates were hung from nails in the basement rafters by their ever-so-long laces. It was up to Marcy and me to get them down. My rail thin big sister lifted me up to unhook each and every pair. One time in so doing, she couldn't hold me long enough to accomplish this task and dropped me, causing one of my fingers to snag on the nail. Well, that incident stopped everything and I was rushed to the hospital emergency room for stitches. I have the momentous scar to this day.

Bandaged but not broken, physically or spiritually, I had extreme directions to keep this gloriously huge white gauze bandage dry. A return to the attending doctor in a week for stitch removal was mandated. In the meantime, I showed off to whomever was available!

Our boggy swamp adventure continued. With the use of mom's kitchen step-stool, getting the skates was much easier ever after. Clothed as before, ice skates replacing boots, we once again trudged to our frozen pond. Gina and Judy learned to ice skate there with us older children as their guides and teachers.

This activity was repeated throughout the winter season and lasted well into February. With below freezing temperatures and the constant accumulation of snow with some dramatic storms, the neighbor kids caught on to our ruckus and often joined in our reverie. However, our "pond" wasn't big enough for all of us. Imagine twenty kids having a "school snow day" and meeting on a twenty foot by 15 foot natural ice pond. It was too crowded. My siblings and I preferred to find something else to do.

After a few winters of being allowed to indulge in this "swamp" play, our privacy on the pond was shattered by more and more neighborhood kids and we moved on to other adventures in the fields. The neighborhood bullies took over and slaughtered the pond, cracked the ice and made it disappear. In one particular kid-attractive field, a tall hill stood, ready to be conquered. A boulder protruded from its center, naturally designed and specific for children to jump off or sled off with a snow-covered ice sheet. Once climbing atop this monster, we could view the neighborhood below, finding one neighbor's house or another. I dubbed this hill "Suicide Hill" and everyone grew to know what we were talking about when we proclaimed "we're going up to Suicide Hill."

There is an enlightened ecstasy of experiencing a snowfall. Once "it's snowing, it's snowing!" had been exclaimed in the house by one of us, a rush to one window or another would redeem the glory. Mom would arm each of us with a brightly colored hard plastic plate and send us outside to catch the flakes. It didn't take long, standing in the cold on the back porch, to be able to view the multitude of various glistening shapes of these ice crystals falling from the sky.

This action of catching-snowflakes with a plate became a tradition. I enjoyed being tenderly and repeatedly kissed by the snowflakes' welcomed arrival. It only takes seconds to experience such sweet, gentle joy! This action caused a warm sensation of delight that has encompassed my childhood time and time again, embedding the memory in my soul.

After such a day of hard, explorative play and a hot supper, it soon became time for bed. "Off to sleep now. Pray for no school tomorrow." I will. Gosh that was fun and I wanted to do that again!

One year, A Mother's Day surprise snowstorm kept us comfortably stranded at our Aunt Betty's and Uncle Johns' house.

You see, Aunt Betty decided to make a celebratory dinner with her three daughters. Unusual as that was my mother was invited with her five kids and Aunt Janet and Uncle Chet with their three kids. It was wonderful, really, and we were all excited when the snow started falling ever-so delicately. After dinner, Uncle John enticed and encouraged all of us to "go outside and play in the snow." Geared up and sharing our older cousins' winter clothes as best as possible, this occasion was quite fun. Even though most of us older kids were put to work to do some shoveling, that task was enjoyably accomplished with about five of us. I imagined that I was filling God's coffee cup with sugar as I shoveled one load after the other. Well, with my Father God being larger than the universe, lots of sugar was needed for his energetic accomplishments!

As this snow fall became relentless, continuing in its accumulation, my mother realized at some point that we were all going to be stuck at Aunt Betty's and Uncle John's house. That wasn't a problem. The problem was that I did not have my insulin. What to do?

The adults concluded that Cousin Mark, Aunt Janet and Uncle Chet's only son, aged about 13 at the time, would hike down the hill to the pharmacy. After a preparatory telephone call to the drug store, Mark was dressed for his hike through the snow for this important and life-saving purchase: the insulin and syringes I needed for that night and the next morning. I remember that my brother wanted to accompany Mark, it could be an adventure after all, but that was discouraged due to his "being too young and we don't have clothes for him."

Poor Mark. He went alone, draped in a heavy snow coat with scarf and hat. I remember anxiously waiting for him to return safely. It seemed to take so long. I sat at the living room window watching for him through the blinding snow, the adults trying to persuade me to get away from the window. I couldn't. I'll never forget the feeling of love and joy I felt for Mark when I saw him trudging up the driveway, package in hand. I honestly didn't care about the insulin, I cared about him. That was the first act of courage and tremendous kindness I had ever been shown.

As evening drew near, each of us were assigned a sleeping spot: extra blankets and pillows lay out on the living room floor or on the cousins' bedroom floor. With my mother's assistance, I was ushered into the bathroom to do what I had to do as far as my nightly injection was concerned. All was at peace. With that done, extra blankets and pillows were pulled out of closets and trunks, thrown to each child who was directed to find a spot on the floor and settle in for the night.

Located in Ayer, Massachusetts, family excursions to the closest military facility/base for supplies were looked forward to, at least to me. With five children to boot in a station wagon (aka: "beach wagon"), shopping was tedious, although well-planned, and less expensive than shopping in the city. Mom knew what needed to be done, what needed to be purchased within her budget, and how to accomplish numerous tasks for her family. Always ahead of her time, she was a multi-tasker before the phrase became popular.

After breakfast, usually on a Saturday in good weather, we were all piled into the green station wagon for the hour-long drive through green and sloping hills of Massachusetts. This task went on for many years. Autumn was the best time for me for such excursions.

A. K. Buckroth

The repeat of New England foliage as it spread across one landscape after another was mesmerizing and relaxing.

The medical facility was visited first, stocking up on prescriptions of insulin, Clinitest tablets, and urine testing strips, Glucagon and most of the necessities to care for *my* diabetes. Glucagon is a powder-to-liquid mixture used with extremely low, convulsive, reactions. Although alcohol swabs were not readily available at that time, mom taught me how to use cotton balls wet with rubbing alcohol that she purchased at the neighborhood drug store.

With this task accomplished, we were off to the 'Commissary' for groceries, shoes, and clothes. Having a well-maintained diabetic diet, never mind a house full of six, was a primary concentration! Not until I was self-supportive did I realize how expensive this disease can be.

Not readily available to the general public, of course, disposable syringes did not immediately replace the glass and metal contraption I had been using. This nasty device, used to give me life, had to be sterilized through boiling every other day. Stored in a covered rectangular metal bowl with matching cover, the components – a glass syringe with metal needle head – was doused in alcohol and hidden in the refrigerator, same spot every day. And every day I greeted it through its freezing cold metallic presence encompassed with the ever-present fumes of rubbing alcohol. This would frighten anyone, let alone a young child. I learned to take care of this device with great respect. I needed it. If I didn't sterilize it, the alcohol in which it lay would become cloudy, smoky looking, dirty - ugly. I wouldn't want to use it. And when I did neglect it to that point, I had to force myself to boil the damn thing before I used it.

I had no choice but to take care of this "metal contraption." Cleanliness was of utmost importance in order to avoid infection, whatever that was! But I was learning, learning, learning. At this time I was 6 – 7 years old and growing to be ever-so-conscious of what I did and did not do. After all, *I* was the one who felt the effects; it was me who felt the repercussions of being self-ignorant, even self-abusive. I often wonder and think about the people effected and affected with and by this disease years and years ago, centuries ago. I've heard of people having to "sharpen their needles." How in the world was this accomplished? It's an ugly visualization to me.

There is a rhyme and reason to the final accomplishment of an insulin injection. First, the contents inside the little glass bottles (vials) full of insulin are "drawn" into the syringe. It was not as easy as it may seem at first. There is a system. The vial(s) need to be rolled between two hands to mix the contents. If two hands are not available, roll the vial(s) on a thigh with one hand or ask someone for help. Then, pull the plunger of the syringe back/down to fill the syringe with air; insert the needle into the vial; push the air-filled syringe with the attached plunger up into the bottle whereas the air replaces the insulin. Carefully watch the tiny lines that are marked on the syringe to indicate how many units are required. Draw back the plunger, wherein insulin will now fill the syringe, replacing the air. Remove syringe from bottle. Tap the syringe lightly in order to cause any air bubbles to float to the tip, closest to the needle. Pushing the plunger lightly will cause the air bubbles to be released from the medication and the syringe. Air bubbles are not a good thing. Some medication may be squirted out at the same time, no big deal. These air bubbles can be released into the air if the syringe is already out of the vial, or they can be released into the insulin vial. It doesn't matter. As long as they are not in the syringe when ready for injection.

Now it is ready to be injected into a specific spot of my body (e.g., buttock, upper thighs, upper arms, lower abdomen). My mother did the subcutaneous injecting and the alcohol swabbing of the chosen area. I was not ready just yet to do it myself. This "life force medication" not only helps make me feel better, but allows me to eat. I like to eat. Insulin is a hormone that assists the body to digest food.

This process wasn't and isn't instantaneous, no siree, especially for a child. I started "drawing" my own insulin when I was six years old but, as mentioned, I did not inject it. Not yet.

To this day, after timing how long it would take my blood glucose level to reach an acceptable level after taking a shot, it has taken the insulin up to 3 hours to bring my blood glucose level to a comfortable level, "comfortable" as in my feeling better.

If the level is above 200, I cannot physically do anything. I feel like a bowl of Jell-o, weak, not well, grouchy, anxious, wanting to be left alone. Below 200, I am happy, chirpy, active, talkative, helpful, personable and feeling pretty.

I can feel coming down, or going up, whichever the case, circumstances, may be. To verify these feelings, I test my blood again. With the use of a "glucometer" (aka: blood machine), this is accomplished 4 – 6 times a day, every day. If I like the results, I hurrah myself, knowing I am able to accomplish something without the fear of becoming fatigued or the fear of becoming shaky with a cold sweat. Those are symptoms of highs or lows.

Three hours is a long time, especially when I've been pressed to accomplish a task. My mind and body just don't seem to work well together when my blood is at a high level. This has led me to believe that I could be resistant to insulin.

Doctors have told me time and time again, "Take your shots at least a half hour before eating/meals." That way, the insulin starts to work before glucose is released through the digestion of food. However, I don't always have that half hour to work with. Too many times I have 'pumped up the jam' while looking at a plate of food. Yes, my digestive process is slowed down, bloating occurs, and I try my best to move, take a walk, to assist myself. However, that is not always the case either. Sometimes, life's situations get in my way. I know people usually do because of *their* wants and demands. I've more often than not put my necessities behind others, as in being a martyr. I hate to admit that but it's true. You see, "people" (aka: friends and family except my mother) forget that I have specific needs. As I have gotten older, I have learned that it is okay to be selfish in the sense of insisting on proper care. For instance, eating at daily scheduled times and exercising twenty minutes after a meal. Actions like these are simple to comprehend but not always respected by others in my company.

And how about the gosh-awful-question that has been asked countless times: "Are you supposed to eat [be eating] that?" Cowering with a feeling of instant guilt, I'll spark up my sarcasm and reply "Sure, why not?" If the inquirer continues on the subject of my eating a certain something, my reply has been "No, but I'm treating myself and will have to give more insulin in order to digest this." There have been too many times I did not know if people were genuinely concerned or just being nosy, pains in the neck! Embarrassment always ensues.

Just as the smell of alcohol or the smell of milk have no comparison, the same with insulin. Even the taste of insulin stands alone. I have found it to be bitter, nasty. I tried it only because I could, out of curiosity. Just like milk tastes like milk and water tastes like water, insulin tastes like nothing but itself. No comparison. And it is original in scent. In fact, there is an oral insulin spray on the market. I have no idea if it's been marketed with a *"New Grape Flavor"* or *"Minty Fresh Taste,"* but I wouldn't even consider myself to be a candidate. The taste and smell is extremely unappealing to me!

Chapter 3
There are others.

Sometime during the course of first grade at St. Mary's in good 'ol Worcester, Massachusetts, a fund drive for the St. Jude Children's Hospital was not only encouraged but practically mandated through my teachers. Hosted by Danny Thomas, all the kids were encouraged to collect money for this institution. At the ages of 8 and 6 respectively, Marcy and I went door-to-door up and down our street to ask for and receive money. I was distinctly under the impression that what I collected was going to buy me a cure for my diabetes. Although that never happened, I continued alongside one or more of my siblings to collect money for this organization throughout the years of my elementary school days. At such a young age, I believed I was helping sick children, including diabetics, to get better somehow.

Danny Thomas. His name and face are forever imprinted on my memory. In later years, his daughter, Marlow Thomas, made a huge impression upon me! You see, she was the first public figure – a movie star! – that I was aware of to have diabetes, to be a diabetic. I was shocked, overwhelmed, dumbfounded to even think that such a beautiful and talented person could have the same disease as I. This news came to me through the *Diabetes Forecast* magazine at the time. As far as I knew, it was the only subscription at the time that was an actual "diabetes updated report." It was *fervently* read in our household with excitement at its arrival in the mail – with my name on it! Receiving it was pure elation. I learned what other kids had to say, becoming familiar with the concept of a pen-pal through that magazine, and actually had a pen-pal. His name was Todd, he lived in Iowa, and he enjoyed building things with his dad. I recall reading one of his letters about his excitement building a tree house with a ten foot ladder.

After learning of Ms. Thomas' being a diabetic, I was heart-broken to read of another actor, *Dan Blocker*, also diabetic. My recollections of him are through a TV character in the late '50's show known as "Bonanza." His character portrayal as *Hoss Cartright* was a physically large, strong and burly man, with a gentleness about him that matched his physique. As a youngster in the '60's, I was attracted to 'Hoss' and looked forward to the weekly show if just for him. Part of that attraction was the unusually tall cowboy hat he wore. Although his obituary does not mention diabetes, he did not die of infamous diabetes complications. I was relieved to learn that!

Speaking of television characters, another stands out especially well for me. It is Ernest Borgnine as character "Commander McHale" in "McHale's" "Navy." As far as I knew, he was not diabetic. It was his physique that greatly reminded me of the father I had due to the Navy involvement. Along with his dark features - tall with dark hair and eyes and a slightly protruding belly, his was the best physical comparison I had as a child to resemble that of my father.

As I grew and continued to read the "Diabetes" magazines that were available, there had been mention of more and more celebrities, movie stars, afflicted with this disease. (e. g., Della Reese, Halle Berry, Wilford Brimley, Delta Burke, Stephen Furst, James Cagney, Dale Evans, Roan Santo (star baseball player), George C. Scott, Kate Smith, Mae West, Nicole Johnson (former Miss America), Jerry Mathers, etc.

I am in total admiration of their coping skills, of their each being able to have an active life, some more active than others from the movies I've watched. I am, once again, in awe if only because I cannot do what they do. Their lives are *extra*-ordinary through their chosen career and its involvements.

The first movie depicting a diabetic character that *I* saw was in *Steel Magnolias*. In essence, it proved to me that diabetes and childbearing/birthing are frightening ordeals for the diabetic and their family members. Quite a tear jerker! Another, *Chocolat*, displayed the harsh reality of repeated insulin injections and the importance of injection rotation as well as staying away from candies – diabetics cannot digest them! In the movie *Panic Room*, a diabetic child acts out the motions of having a convulsion in one horrific scene. However, treating the convulsion with insulin is definitely _not_ the thing to do. That was misleading to the general public proving to me that diabetes remains misunderstood with the media. In a convulsive state, insulin would bring coma and death to a diabetic.

Other films – *Nothing in Common*, *Reversal of Fortune*, and *Regarding Henry* - portray poignant relations with diabetes through diabetic characters, but they just don't hit the nail on the head, at least not for me.

Musicians effected with this disease as far as I have learned from my research for this writing have been Bret Michaels ("Poison), Tommy Lee ("Motley Crue"), Waylon Jennings (country singer), Dizzy Gillespie (jazz trumpeter), Ella Fitzgerald (jazz vocalist), B. B. King (rhythm and blues star), Mick Fleetwood ("Fleetwood Mac"), Johnny Cash (country), Syd Barrett ("Pink Floyd"), Miles Davis (jazz), Meat Loaf (singer), Jerry Garcia ("Grateful Dead"), Peggy Lee (50's singer), Carol Channing (singer/actress), and so many, many more.

Now I read and hear of actresses, actors, and musicians' children and grandchildren being affected! This fact is unsobering to me, unsettling. It seems like the world is becoming covered in this stuff, diabetes, and it's just getting worse! It's endless.

A few years back, I either heard about or read about, as usual, a television show about diabetes. My television guide never displayed such a show. I blamed this on not having an extensive and expensive cable channel. However, through an internet Google search, I typed in "Diabetes Television" and it came up. Known as "dLifeTV," the show does air at certain times depending on which region of the country you live in. It advertises as "Information, Inspiration and Connection for Your Diabetes Life."

My Diabetic Soul

The St. Jude's Hospital collection went on for many years, most, if not all, of my elementary school days with the inclusion of our younger siblings once they were old enough to walk with us. Always in a cold, New England fall, mom bundled us up after supper, remaining in our school uniforms, to accomplish this task. Not only did we represent St. Mary's but we represented the onslaught of diabetes. I knew the nuns at school would be happy with our booty. Praise was appreciated and well heard, incentive enough for me to do it again. Simple.

Well, the neighbors, all of them on that street, got to know us pretty well. It wasn't long before doors were opened in welcome and dollars and change poured into our manila collection envelopes. Surprisingly, we never did receive a gift, a prize, some type of incentive that is offered these days to children in their elementary schools when they collect a certain amount of money, the most money of their peers. Collections were done out of the goodness of our hearts with a Christian attitude. We did it because it was a good thing – a pain in the neck – but a good thing nonetheless. It brought hope to this disease. Hope of a cure.

Novena to St. Jude

> *Most holy Apostle, St. Jude, faithful servant and friend of*
> *Jesus, the Church honors and invokes you universally, as*
> *the patron of difficult cases,*
> *of things almost despaired of.*
> *Pray for me, I am so helpless and alone.*
> *Intercede with God for me that He bring*
> *Visible and speedy help.*
> *Come to my assistance in the great need*
> *That I may receive the consolation and help of heaven*
> *In all my necessities, tribulations, and Suffering,*
> *particularly [with diabetes].*
> *And that I may praise God with you*

And all the saints forever. I promise, O Blessed St. Jude, to be ever mindful of this great favor granted me by God to always honor you as my special and powerful patron, and to gratefully encourage devotion to you. Amen.

To this day, St. Jude's Children's Hospital is a thriving enterprise affecting childhood illnesses and diseases of all kinds with effervescent hope! St. Jude is a spiritual and personal ally. I faithfully wear a medallion of St. Jude, patron saint of the hopeless, a saint acknowledged for terminal cases, along with my Medic Alert medallion. After all, I am terminal. I wear both medallions with pride as an acceptance to myself of myself, but to allow others some peace of mind.

Managing diabetes *in school* had not become a headline until October 8, 2003, to be exact. The keyword is "managing." In California, Assembly Bill 942 was passed to allow diabetic students to be able to use their managing supplies (e.g., glucose meters) and medications (insulin injections, glucose tablets) anywhere on school grounds as opposed to having to go to the nurses' office and/or principal's office. Of course, this depends upon the comprehension level of the diabetic student regarding his/her knowledge of self-care. Self-care is *very* important and gained through knowledge, grown through experience.

"I long to accomplish a great and noble task, but it is my chief duty to accomplish small tasks as if they were great and noble."
~ Helen Keller ~

Due to the aforementioned fundraiser, we kids became familiar with the neighbors. This was a gateway of happiness through familiarity *especially* once Halloween came around.

Chapter 4
Tempestuous, tempting holidays.

Oh, Glorious Autumn!

Cooler temperatures and windy weather invite numerous tree leaves to shed from their boughs and branches. Shaded and vivid colors of yellow from the oaks, red from the maples, with splotches of purple and varying shades of the primary color palette take over the living earth at this season of every year. This is my favorite time of year. There is a certain passion among the colors as they fly through the air, on every street and territory disguised as leaves. Tourists continually arrive to see the spectacular foliage that peaks in mid-October, enjoying New England hospitality.

Through the harvesting of cabbages at this time of year in Massachusetts, mom would take all of us to a family farm in Oxford, Massachusetts. She would choose the largest head of cabbage she could find. In a huge bin full of cabbages, she would roll one over another and another in search of the perfect cabbage. The largest ones were found at the bottom of the bin and she needed help to get one out. Heck, it was always bigger than a bowling ball! Along with the seasons' pumpkins of which one was purchased for each of us, she would also purchase at least two shopping bags full of Macintosh apples. The car ride home was full of munchkins munching apples and the smell of freshly unearthed vegetables and the dirt on our shoes from mulling about the farm.

The main purpose of the extra special cabbage was to make *gołąbkis* (stuffed cabbage leaves). Mother did this by first preparing a ground beef mixture of white rice and spices. Once the cabbage was thoroughly boiled in the hugest pot she had, it had to be cooled for the next process. Hours went by. When ready, Marcy and I would tenderly separate the soft cabbage leaves with our little fingers, placing the wet leaves aside.

Mother would hand me pieces of limp cabbage to eat, the leaves that couldn't be used because they were either too small, or she noticed me drooling. "You can eat this Andrea. Cabbage has no calories," she told me. And I did, of course.

Mother would then take a handful of the beef mixture, place it on a cabbage leaf, and fold it ever-so-delicately so that each gołąbki was tightly wrapped and sealed, something like an overstuffed envelope. Using the same huge pot in which the cabbage was originally boiled, two or three cabbage leaves were placed in the pots' bottom. This was done to prevent burning any of the dozens of gołąbkis that were placed in that pot. Then they were boiled all together. The scent alone was – is – deliciously unmistakable! Served with slices of dark rye bread with butter and a tall glass of cold milk, this meal is completely satisfactory. This was a big favorite in our house!

A lot of preparation went into this meal, lasting into leftovers that were looked forward to in coming days. Many of these gołąbkis were placed into a plastic food storage container for freezing.

The Polish diet is very bland yet healthy and safe as far as calories are concerned. Kielbasa is boiled, peirogis are boiled, chicken is boiled for soup or typically baked, beets are boiled for burak zupa (beet soup), and you already know about the cabbage. It took me a long time as an adult to adjust my taste buds to spicy foods. Fried foods were unavailable in my mother's house. It was very rare that I indulged eating fried foods if only because I did not like them. Therefore, through my Polish upbringing, my diabetes and I have had a healthy start in life! I consider this factor as not only a great advantage, but a blessing as well.

Halloween soon arrived with anxious excitement and creative preparations and decorations all through the city!

Our house was no different. Inclusive with the carved pumpkins that each of us intrinsically carved in detail and set outside on the front steps with a candle lit inside each one, our school artwork was scotch-taped on windows to display the holiday spirit. Orange construction paper presented hand cut-outs of pumpkins; white construction paper was used to portray a ghostly figure or two; black construction paper was used to portray cut-outs of witches and bats. Color crayons further helped to display facial images, with or without blood. Ahh, the creative minds of children!

Our costume preparations were the most fun for our trick-or-treating event. There was no 'running to the store to *buy* a costume.' No, no, no. Mom was greatly creative, encouraging, and patient with this endeavor. We were allowed to go through her things – all her things including clothes, jewelry, hats, make-up, and what have you, and anything else we kids could find – in order to 'dress up' and disguise ourselves. Oh, there were limits of course, but just being allowed to rummage through her things was magnificent in itself! Imagine a family of four or five children (Judy wasn't old enough yet), costumed to the nines, knocking on your door with goody bags (pillowcases were the best) outstretched! It was hilarious. Because of mothers' encouragement, I still look forward to this "holiday" every year.

The best costume I recall was my brother being a mummy. He got the idea from the infamous 1960's movie entitled "The Mummy." He gathered all the ace bandages he could muster. Mom kept them for her sore, tired legs. Imagine a 10-year old boy wrapped in ace bandages from head to foot. It was marvelous and the funniest thing I ever did see! Toward the end of this particular trick-or-treating event, his bandages started coming off, actually making him look more eerie. I remember laughing and laughing, trying to help him tuck one end of a bandage in to where it had loosened, only to have another one pop out. It was hilarious! I fell on the ground laughing with tears in my eyes. He was upset. I could tell he was getting frustrated. The only thing he wore under all these Ace bandages was a pair of BVD's (shortened nick-name of boys' underwear stands for Bradley, Voorhees & Day, the New York City firm that initially manufactured underwear of this name for both men and women. BVD is now only for men. It was founded in 1876 and named for

A. K. Buckroth

its three founders. (**Wikipedia [the Internet Free] Encyclopedia**).

Once inside our house, he ripped those things off as soon as he could, swearing he'd never do that again, and continued to enjoy his candy collection.

It wasn't until a later age, about the time when I was twelve that real scary, bad, things began to happen through the unlawful and horrible tainting of Halloween treats. Our first experience was a razor blade in an apple. From then on, the candy bags had to be checked and re-checked. Imagine having to do that for 5 kids!

Nevertheless, I wasn't shy when it came to eating some of that stuff. Oh no. My siblings did not witness this sneaky cheating. Otherwise I would have been chastised to the mountains and grounded and probably banned from any further participation for the rest of my life! You see, my manipulations caused my older sister to walk ahead with the younger kids while I carried the rear, purposely. While dusk turned to dark, I gluttonously indulged in many a forbidden sweet. I almost hate to admit it but my favorite chocolates bars became Almond Joy and Butterfingers, the little ones, so it didn't seem so bad. But, when I ate too many as is prone to happen with any child, I became ill. It wasn't so much the stomach ache, but my blood sugar was on top of the moon!

I didn't need to take a urine test to know that I messed up. Bloated stomach, sleepy with lethargy, I needed insulin. So I took it. I knew how. I first learned how to give myself an insulin shot at the age of six through my young involvements with the Clara Barton Birthplace Camp (now known as *The Barton Center*) for diabetic girls. Using only the clear, "Regular" kind because it was "fast-acting," it still took a few hours until I felt better, was better.

In the meantime, the "Sugar-free Halloween Fairy" came to visit our house while we were out. My mother placed a special purchase of sugar-free goodies under a pillow or atop the bureau chiding me to see if I found anything unusually special.

Gosh, that was gloriously thoughtful. That type of heartfelt kindness is rekindled to this day.

And the "Halloween Fairy" along with the "Valentine's Fairy," the

"Easter Bunny," and whatever character was implicated during certain and specific times of each year was an implication that there existed diabetic characters of each holiday genre. There were some that were just plain sugar-free, like me, and they knew where I lived and left me treats!

What "real" holiday follows Halloween? Thanksgiving!

As soon as the Halloween decorations were packed away, the Thanksgiving turkey pictures, the festive tablecloth and more school creations took their place. The all ready purchased and to-be-baked-turkey was nestled in its frozen sanctuary in the cellar freezer; the sack of potatoes rested near the sacks of apples, also in the coolness of the cellar.

The night before Thanksgiving, a certain number of apples were brought upstairs first. Pies were going to be made! Marcy and I were in charge of peeling the apples, slicing them, and setting them aside in a big bowl. Yes, there was more than one occasion when either of us cut a finger and had to attend to it. While we were occupied with this task in the kitchen, mother kept the younger ones busy in another part of the house. I don't know what they were all doing, but I didn't care because I had to concentrate on peeling the apples. There were a lot them!

In our house, this holiday was celebrated with not only regular, sugared apple pies, but also with sugar-free apple pies. There were less sugar-free pies (usually two in all) than the regular ones because I was the only one to eat them *for a time*. Actually, I got bored with them after a while and often had to throw one away due to its having turned green.

I recall being 8 years old when my mother taught me how to make and bake a sugar-free pie. It's so simple, really. There are the regular ingredients, but no sugar. Because apples are naturally sweetened, the addition of cinnamon is – voila – a sugar-free pie! I continue the tradition to this day, marveling at non-diabetics who marvel at my sugar-free creations.

The morning of any Thanksgiving Day, there came a time to peel the potatoes. It was usually Marcy and I, again, to go downstairs, count out and carry up about 5 potatoes each. This of course was for the mashed potatoes. She and I peeled those and the carrots, which prompted a peeled finger or two that would heed a break from kitchen duty. Fresh cranberries were washed and steamed for me; regular cranberry jelly was set out for the others. Black olives and a variety of pickles were appropriately and neatly placed in the proper crystal-ware platter. According to my diet, one olive is worth one pat of butter due to its caloric fat content. That meant no freely eating those. The pickles I could eat all I wanted.

The table was formally and beautifully set using mother's better china and her silver dinnerware. Crystal bowls and glasses complimented each other at each place setting of six. Cloth napkins were laid at each place setting with the proper arrangement of the proper utensils. Larger crystal bowls were placed in the living room on the coffee table full of unshelled nuts of every variety in existence with appropriate nut-cracking tools; another bowl was filled to the brim with fresh and colorful fruits such as tangerines, grapes of every color with a variety of apples, figs, and dates. Sumptuousness can be gorgeous with the significance of gratitude!

Dinnertime, finally. Having foregone my mid-morning snack in order to partake in this offered and prepared higher-carbohydrate dinner, I was hungry, famished. The dark meat of a baked turkey was and remains my favorite. I do not mind gnawing on a thigh bone or a wing, as long as the skin is crunchy. Although I would take a small portion of the mashed potatoes, I preferred and prefer stuffing. Mother's was made with bread crumbs, celery, mushrooms and onions. I would rather forego butter or margarine in order to have gravy. I heeded what I knew about food substitutions, as expressed on page 26, without any unjust consequences. Actually, I was, and am, the better for it.

Christmas Eve was more of a celebration than Christmas Day in our house. As a family, we celebrated the *Wilia* (the "W" pronounced as an English "V") Supper. "This holiday is preceded by a period of four weeks during which fast is observed on Wednesdays, Fridays and Saturdays. Strict fast is observed throughout the day before Christmas, and in the evening the Wilia Supper is served. This is a feast to commemorate the birth of the God Child."

"The Supper itself differs from other evening meals in that the number of courses is fixed at seven, nine or eleven; and in no case must there be an odd number of people at the table. A lighted candle in the window symbolizes the hope that the God Child, in the form of a stranger, may come to share the Wilia Supper, and an extra place is set at the table for the expectant guest. This belief stems from the ancient Polish adage, 'Guest in the home is God in the home." **(Sokolowski, Marie and Jasinski, Irene. Treasured Polish Recipes for Americans, © 1948.)**

As far as fasting for me was concerned, I was excused because of my diabetes. No matter what holiday or occasion it was, I did not have to 'fast.' My mother and I went to the parish rectory and she explained to the priest the reasoning behind this request. It was granted before my First Holy Communion in 1965.

Mom slaved by herself the whole day preparing for this dinner. That meant that we kids had to stay out of the way. It was up to us older ones, Marcy and I, to keep the younger ones, and ourselves, occupied. If mom needed help in the kitchen, usually with cleaning the shrimp, Marcy or I would volunteer. That way we would get an advanced taste of what was to come.

Many days in advance, specialty food items were purchased. Shopping sprees to the Polish specialty food section of Worcester remains on Water Street to this day. Being acquainted with the area, three to four stores on one block usually had everything that mom needed. She served pickled herring, a white rice ring with steamed shrimp, cauliflower, mushroom soup, pierogi, and baked sauerkraut in butter. I have no idea the caloric content of any of these courses, and I did not – and do not – care. If my mother said it was okay to eat them, I ate them. Yes, dessert was served as well. This was Jesus' birthday cake that consisted of an Angel Food cake laced with strawberries and whipped cream. Angel Food Cake was the best-to-be-found cake/pastry for the diabetic in our house. A typical, non-diabetic household would have the Polish *chruściki*, deep fried dough with confectioner's sugar sprinkled on top. Those were a no-no in our house! What we had was all so very delicious and looked forward to every Christmas Eve!

Before sitting down to the table, we each broke off a piece of the traditional *Opłatek*, "a thin unleavened wafer like the altar bread in Church. Stamped with the figures of the God Child, the Blessed Mary, and the Holy Angels. It is known as the bread of love." Breaking off a small piece of this 6-inch by 3½-inch wafer, we exchanged a blessing with everyone present. This meant each of us, one-by-one, was to walk around the steaming and beautifully set dinner table to greet my mother, and each other. They did the same. The main purpose of this tradition is to "remind participants of the importance of Christmas, God, and Family."
(Wikipedia [the Internet Free] Encyclopedia.)

For example, I have simply said to my mother "Thank you for your cooking skills." To my brother or sisters, I would wish them well in an upcoming venture, event and/or plan.

With the six of us, together, we were safe. A candle was lit, resting in the center of the kitchen dinner table with its flame remaining ignited throughout the meal.

Church "processions" were the norm back then at St. Mary's. As mentioned, the Church affiliated with that school is "Our Lady of Częstochowa" after a city in Poland. I do not doubt that these ceremonial Catholic traditions are continued. Before the Church's' specific *Christmas processional* and after *Wilia*, the house was full of preparedness activities. For instance, my hair was set in "pin-curls" for a curled coif. Because my hair was always long and stick-straight, mom would spend hours winding a strand of my hair around her fingers and clamp it to my scalp with a bobby-pin. I must have had a hundred bobby pins attached to my head! The effect was to produce curls, long, wavy, luxuriant and attractive curls. It worked – for a little while. "Bologna curls" were tried using strands of cloth but my hair never did hold a curl. That process was not only tedious, but extremely uncomfortable.

Year after year through elementary school, one or two of my siblings and I would participate in these elaborate affairs with many of our older and younger school mates. Processions were literal traditions, encompassing ideals of Catholicism and its respectful beliefs through pageants of play-acting according to the respected months' biblical occasion. One year, during fourth or fifth grade, I was asked to portray the Virgin Mary herself for the Christmas Eve procession. My responsibility was to carry the plaster infant doll, Jesus, down the aisle to the altar and stay sitting there throughout the two-hour Mass while holding that doll. The doll itself was old, tarnished, having a chip on its body. Not what I thought Baby Jesus should look like at all! Quietly sufficing my appall, I went forward with the practiced requirements of this dramatization. A boy depicting the saintly "Joseph" character was already at the altar. For the life of me, I cannot remember who that was.

The month of May celebrated the Holy Days of the Virgin Mother, Mary. As my friend, Ricky, recalls, "the May Procession was held on the first Sunday in May with the prefect of the high school sodality, a female high school senior, having been chosen as the "May Queen." She was required to wear a wedding dress, a crown of roses, and referred to as 'Mary, the Queen of Heaven.'

"Lots of little children," continues Ricky, "passed out and vomited in the hot sun. Parents took home-movies that 40 years later would serve as blackmail material. Oh, it was a wonderful time in life!" True sarcasm.

My mother, along with the other "chosen ones" parents, tailored ritualistic preparations with each of her children for such events. This always began with the purchasing of fabric and thread, but not always a pattern. Mom made the requisite 'costumes' for each of us for each of these processions. Always white, the color symbolized the state of virginity as it continues to do in this country.

They were beautiful! Always and everyone was beautiful! After all, my mother has beautiful children! And her beautiful talents as a designer and seamstress were bestowed upon her children.

Every holiday held a procession with standing-room-only in the Church with people having to park blocks away in order to attend. Christmas and Easter have been the most lavish affairs in this parish. While all that pomp and glory and practice was going on, one very important thing had to be included – sugar! Yep, in each palm of my little hand, inside the customary white cloth gloves, I held and carried a packet of sugar. This was "just in case" I had a "reaction." As explained earlier, such a thing is synonymous to the term "hypoglycemic reaction," or "incident."

Well, I don't recall ever having to eat the stuff. More often than not it melted in my hand anyway, causing me to throw the sticky paper away. If there were no packets available, mom required me to use sugar cubes. Gosh, that was uncomfortable and not a pretty sight as it bulged through my gloves but it was all we had.

We got through it along with all the other processions without too much of a scene. I was very happy to have been of service. If not for the attention due to one or another of my home-made dresses, nobody knew a thing about the sugar!

Christmas Day brought the opportunity to eat the ever-loved sugar-free cookies that mom baked yesterday, *before* our lavish Wilia. In preparation for this sugar-free baking, the table was cleared after the sugar baking stuff was done. No traces of that ingredient were going to touch any surface of this sugar-free creation!

Flour and the other dry ingredients were mixed (always causing a mess), an egg or two was beaten, maybe broken, maybe rolled across the kitchen floor, and walnuts were chopped and dropped. Looking back, mom learned everything necessary, I mean EVERYTHING, in order take care of me. And she was strict! However, part of this knowledge included such home-made treats in my diet. There was nothing on the grocery store shelves as far as sugar-free baked cookies were concerned, not until *many* years later. I'll say again, my diet was stringent! Food portions were measured and counted to maintain a specific and certain daily caloric intake. For instance, 15 grapes or 15 cherries were an allowable dessert at any one time; 15 potato chips if those were available; 1 small apple or orange; 5 saltines equal one piece of bread; etc. *Stringency with caution* amounted to self-discipline throughout my childhood!

Substitution of an edible item meant doing without something else. Substitutions were and are one of the daily rules for me and my diet. It was a balancing of my daily caloric intake. With that in mind, choices had to be made. Well, of course I went for the cookies or the pie, doing without a full glass of milk or a full serving of mashed potatoes. That was okay. That's the way it was – and is today. Special attention is just fine with me! It's the gaining of weight that can become a problem. I know it's due to not paying attention, becoming lax in my stringency; a lack of self-discipline. This disease has been tiring!

I'd like to make a special note regarding all store-bought, sugar-free treats. They cause gas. Yep. Made with sugar alcohols, diuretics if you will, please be forewarned of gassiness and bloating when eating sugar-free products! Sugar alcohols are sorbitol, maltitol and xylitol. In fact, to prove my theory of gassiness to unbelievers, I've had many comical opportunities to share sugar-free treats with non-diabetics. I made a believer out of them! My most recent finding was a bagful of sugar-free Baby Ruth chocolate bars. I couldn't believe it! However, I am speechlessly delighted in just knowing that they exist!

Why Sugar-Free Foods Have a 'Laxative Effect'
By Kristen McNutt, PhD., JD

> *"Like fiber, sugar replacers are only slightly digested – or not at all.*

> *"Therefore, [the] most low-digestible carbohydrate that is eaten is not absorbed. The body's normal response to*

unabsorbed carbohydrates is simply to dilute them by pulling water across the intestine lining into the upper part of the intestine. When low-digestible carbohydrates move into the large intestine, most of that water moves back in the opposite direction. Depending on how much water flowed in and out, stools might be unchanged, soft or loose. This is why low-digestible carbohydrates are sometimes used to relieve constipation.

Some bacteria that live in the large intestine can "eat" low-digestible carbohydrates, and they use this type of carbohydrate for their own growth. After they have eaten, gases and short fatty acids remain. That's why beans, fiber and other sources of low-digestible carbohydrates may cause an increase of gas. Recent research shows that some of the short fatty acids promote intestinal health. Furthermore, two sugar replacers (isomalt and lactitol) have been found to stimulate the growth of "good" bacteria in the intestine.

"The possibility of loose stools and gas can be reduced by eating only small quantities of low-digestible carbohydrate. Give your body some time to adjust to digesting these foods." **McNutt, Kristen, PhD., JD. Diabetes Interview, February 2004, Issue 139, Volume 13, Number 2.**

Well, thank you very much, Dr. McNutt. This answers my questions and decades of eating, often gluttonously, so so many sugar-free treats. Now people will believe me!

Chapter 5
"This little light of mine, I'm gonna let it shine..."
...a long, long time.

Summers at the Clara Barton Birthplace Camp in North Oxford, Massachusetts, were the highlight of my childhood.

Recalling at the age of six the first time my mother brought me there I was overwhelmed and speechless. There were actually other children – my age and size – that had diabetes too! They were walking around with their parents and brothers and sisters just as I was! Introductions were made and friendships were immediately established if you were going to be in the same cabin as I! Immediately nicknamed "Andy" with my approval that is who I became, "Andy."

I was excited. "Elated" is probably a better word. You see, a non-diabetic person has to realize the queerness of this disease in 1964. Ostracized by classmates at a young age, I began a life of secrecy as mentioned earlier. Not only did people not know of my diabetes, but it never did imprint itself in label form on any part of my body. Nor was I an unusual shade of color. Therefore, I appeared and seemed to be a happy, beautifully normal, healthy child.

Within these neatly lawned grounds, there were *others like me*! Kids! My age!

The history behind this camp is short but succinct, beginning in 1932. Clara Barton, a well-acknowledged Civil War nurse, was born here in 1821. Ms. Barton's claim to fame was her founding the American Red Cross organization through her compassionate humanitarianism. Being a Universalist, her Church purchased the 96 acres of land for use for inner-city youths. With Dr. Elliott P. Joslin's dedication to diabetic children as far back as 1921, these combined efforts and knowledge led to the creation of The Clara

Barton Birthplace Camp. I am honored to have been a part of this
endeavor. (**Liz Sonneborn.** <u>**Clara Barton Founder, American Red
Cross**</u>; © 1992. **Barton Center for Diabetes Education. Wikipedia, the
free [internet] encyclopedia.**)

My first year there, I was assigned to a twin bunk in one of five
cottages. This one was called "Squirrels Nest." This cottage
allowed eight girls aged six and seven, to sleep and keep their
things. All the cabins were basic and hollow wooden structures
without foundations, having three rooms each. Two larger rooms at
opposite ends of the cabin housed four twin bunk beds for four girls
and their belongings; the middle space housed two twin bunk beds,
one for each of two counselors and their belongings. All eight girls
and two councilors became team members, buddies, pals, and
caretakers of each other in this small, colorful learning and happy
place. We were to live together for three weeks amidst nature.

This was my first experience with summer camp and being away
from home. I was excited and happy to be away. Eight more
summers were to follow. Each of these summers housed me and
other diabetic girls of the same age. As I grew, I was able to
experience similar comforts of cabin lodgings inside "Seaside
Lagoon," "Wind-in-the-Pines," "Lakeside," "Rainbow Ridge," or
"Shang-Ri-La." Purposely placed among the lush green acres of the
area and surrounding the camp's pond, I shared my young life in
many of these cabins with exploitive and explosive energy. Years
later as an older camper, a teenager, I was housed with others of my
age in tents on wooden platforms across the road and up a long rock
lined dirt path in the woods.

Each camper was supplied with her very own trunk specifically in
tow with the 'summer wardrobe at camp,' following the directions
of an 'inventory list.' Trunks were neatly kept at the foot of each
bunk-bed. However, these trunks always held much more than a
wardrobe. Consider the special quilt patched by a mother or
grandmother; or the new supply of stationery with stamps and pens
and pencils; pictures of other family members; stuffed animals and

favorite dolls of comfort; maybe a few books so as not to forget the school book reports due in the fall. Packable love represented by endearing objects.

Awakened each morning at seven o'clock to the trumpeting sound of the American militaristic revelry was performed by a councilor, Debby. Campers – *all* campers – were trained to quickly grab their assigned "pee pots" and proceed to the restroom for a "fasting glucose test." We were instantly mobilized!

Conveniently stored under each child's bunk for safekeeping, the precise purpose of a "pee pot" was for glucose testing via a urine specimen before each meal. This determined the amount of insulin required for each young body to balance her food intake, insulin amount, and the scheduled exercise programs.

The chilly morning air awakened and encouraged this responsibility to our selves. Covered in goose bumps, the sparkling morning dew remained asleep on the grass carpet until all the children clomped over it to the lavatory. Sleepy heads had no choice but to awaken. Parading through the lawn with dews' heavy wetness as it sparkled in the sunrise was enough to keep me alert and careful not to slip. It was cold and wet! Oftentimes I wore my slippers during this march because they were ready and waiting for me aside my bunk. My tennis shoes just took too long to find, put on, and tie the laces. Each and every camper was assigned a clear plastic "pee pot." We had to carefully balance those pots, and ourselves, to accomplish this first task of the day.

The "pee pot" was essentially used for urine glucose testing four times each day during the duration of her stay. The design of the pee pots were exactly those containers used for potty training little kids – a hard, sturdy, clear plastic container with a handle for ease in dumping out the contents in a toilet. I know. I had one at home along with my baby sister who was being potty-trained.

Imagine eight 6 year-old girls awakened at 7:00am, in slippers and pajamas, trying ever so carefully to scurry across the wet lawn to the large lavatory building, bringing their morning "fasting" samples for glucose testing. Not all made it, having slipped in the dew or tripped over themselves, spilling the contents. We often bumped into each other, our eyes on the containers and not on who was in front of us. "Eeck, you just spilled on me!" was often heard. "You poured some on my slippers!" cried another. Mayhem with bad feelings occurred with the councilors having to step up and keep everyone calm and orderly to accomplish this task. We were encouraged to hurry because the older kids were coming for the same reason, with the same type of containers, and they did not like little kids in their way!

This accidental sloshing and oftentimes splattering of urine by these half-awakened walking youths did not halt time for embarrassment. This was a daily routine. Four times a day – before breakfast, lunch, supper, and bedtime snack. Occasionally, a child was required to test more often due to the brittleness of her disease, the adjustment of a new routine or a new type of insulin, and/or another of many of life's emotional quandaries. All this was taken into consideration for the days' insulin amount and requirement. It had to be. Growing pangs, puberty, and etceteras were taken into consideration depending upon the specific phase of life. It was your life, your body, and you had to learn to grow with it, live with it, and take care of it.

There were hundreds of pee pots shelved in this huge, colorless and windowless restroom during any one day. At night, before scrambling under bed covers, each child returned her personal pee pot under her bunk in her appropriate cabin. I always made sure mine was kept under my bunk next to my slippers and all ready for the next mornings' fasting.

Once inside this cold, grey, concrete slab building, two or three older girls were seated behind a metal table top built out of one wall. They watched and heard all of this commotion each morning. These characters may have changed but the lingo remained the same. "Watch it!" one girl would scream before getting a pee pot spilled on her. "Be careful!" Due to the outside grassy wetness having been brought inside by many pairs of shoes, the lavatory floor became a slippery, sloshy mess. It was the responsibility of these two or three older girls to label each child's pot with the child's name in heavy black magic marker. Then they took samples with an eye dropper device, placing the sample in a clear glass vial and dropping in a Clinitest tablet. I never waited for my glucose results. I was too hungry and wanted to get up the hill to the mess hall for breakfast. But first, I had to return to the cabin to get dressed.

One-gallon, clear plastic, 24-hour urine bottles also took up space above the pee pot shelves. These were for the use of collecting any campers' urine over a period of 24 hours to ensure proper kidney function. Those large bottles were an implied sign: if another camper had to use one of those, it meant she could have the first signs of the complication of kidney disease. No, I did not know what a kidney was or what it did, but I overheard enough conversations that a person's kidney was very important and had to be taken care of.

That lavatory building often stank! If the lingering smell of urine and Magic Marker didn't wake you up, then the replacement scent of bleach and antiseptic sure would! I experienced these scents every day. The lavatory's smell of chlorine and disinfectant mixed with Magic Marker fumes rekindles memories.

Staying three weeks at a time for the next nine summers of my life, a new "pee pot" container greeted me every year, always the same design. There was nothing creative about them! Over the course of time, the one I used at home was replaced every two or three years. If the plastic started yellowing and cracking, that was a sure sign that it was on its way to the trash.

On the camp grounds was the original barn – still standing - and used on the weekends for the campers' dances and other activities popular to the time. Although my mother taught me how to polka, that was inappropriate for the pop music at camps' social dances. Therefore, I learned how to dance by watching the older kids and councilors dance. The older ones would encourage the younger ones to dance with them, showing them how to coordinate their feet, arms, hips and whole body to music. One summer, a donated trampoline was set up in this barn for all of us campers to enjoy. That was my first and only experience of playing on a trampoline. It was fun jumping and flying through the air while kicking and twisting before landing in a bounce on the trampoline.

In my early teen years, aged 13 – 14 as a camper, a group of us had a sarcastic saying to "normal" people, usually adults: "Can't you see I'm green?! You should know that diabetics are green!!" Budding New England sarcasm among budding teenage girls is a wonderful learning experience, however rude to those whom are not in on the conversation. Later known as "peer pressure," I remain glad to have been a part of it!

The summation of life at Clara Barton Camp (CBC) encouraged a positive outlook toward a fuller life for juvenile diabetics. It is now called "The Barton Center for Diabetes Education, Inc., Inspiring Children, Empowering Families."

Upon returning home one summer, my mother was excited about a new innovation she had learned about called "destrostix." Purposefully used for the testing of sugar levels in a persons' urine, their container was comparable to the container size of swimming pool and/or hot tub water testing strips. Yes, they had to be peed upon. Well, I did not like that at all. Having to hold a strip in mid-stream caused me to have too many accidents where I ended up peeing on my fingers. Forget it!

When it came to camp life, it was really an escape for me. It was also acceptable in the sense that my mother greatly encouraged my going away for three weeks. My brother and sisters knew it was important for me to go away to learn about myself with this disease even though they were so young. They would see me soon enough with stories to tell and share about all the wonderful things I learned. They would meet my new friends at the end of three weeks and be ever-so-glad for me to get home once again.

Ahh, what a life! However, my personal happiness was overshadowed by the disappearance of my father in my life, during this same time period. This was my father whom I would not see again until I was 18 years old. That was part of the drama I mentioned earlier as well as it being another story. Bad dreams awoke me many nights in tears, my camp counselors thinking I was having a convulsion when I was dreaming about my father being lost. He didn't know where I was! I didn't know where he was! How was he going to find me? How was he going to know that I was all right? My concerns were negated, swept up in a world of day-to-day survival.

Those three weeks of each year from July to August I spent in an environment of a grassed carpet hugged with trees and the awakening smell of pine. To this day, that natural fragrance of pine with its beauty remains a pleasant one, enlightening wonderful memories. The smell of pine instantaneously brings me back to camp.

Each glorious day was a learning experience. Not only did I learn about the disease in my body, but I also learned that diabetes wasn't just <u>my</u> disease. Other kids had it. These other kids had to do the same routine each day. The same routine as I did! How awesome! These other kids had to take insulin shots and pee in a cup and share living space and eat at the same table with rigorous dietary needs. We all learned to sing songs such as "This Little Light of Mine," "Abbalaba Gabbalaba Goobala Beesay," "Oh Mister Moon," and too many more. My compatriots reading this book can attest to the other songs, I'm sure.

With the lavatory task accomplished for the time being, I and all of my new friends scurried as quickly as possible back to our cabins to quickly dress for the day and then proceed to the infirmary for our morning insulin shots. As breakfast was diligently served at 8:00am in the mess hall each morning, dressing quickly and getting your shot was a prerequisite to eating.

It was there, in the CBC camp ground infirmary where I learned to give myself an insulin shot. Having to climb a set of stairs to gain entrance into this facility, I was always greeted by one or two nurses. You could pick them out immediately with their white uniforms and white shoes. At that age, I knew all too well what a nurse looked like.

Similar to my cabin, this building also had no foundation and rested upon six stilts. The nurses' sleeping quarters were in the back, to the left of the entrance. To the right, there was a narrow hall where I could see two other rooms, one on the left and one on the right. In the center inside the entry way, there were shelves and shelves of medical supplies lining the walls: boxes of syringes, boxes of alcohol swabs, boxed gauzes and band-aids of varying shapes and sizes, first aid kits, refrigerators, and everything a medical staff would need to do whatever they were required to do.

A part of every morning routine, after urine testing and dressing, involved every single child to march up the steps to the infirmary, state her name, be handed a filled syringe, and inject herself. Standing behind what I remember as a very long table, the two nurses greeted me and asked me "Are you ready, Andy?" This table was full of needles (filled insulin syringes). There were many of them, lined up one after the other with a name at each needle. One of the nurses picked up one of the syringes saying "Here you go, Andy. Have a seat right over there and I'll help you give it to yourself." I knew this was coming. I had heard a few of the other girls exclaim how they had given themselves their shots and how it was no big deal.

Not knowing how to do this beforehand, one of the nurse's had been doing it for me. However, that was short lived. There came that day when I was told "no breakfast until you give yourself a shot!" Yikes! The pressure was on. I was told to decide where I wanted to put it, "maybe your thigh would be easiest. Sit over here," the nurse said.

I sat across from the doorway, thinking of a way to escape. I did not want to do this! Tutored beforehand on the process with the use of an orange, I pinched some thigh meat with my left hand, held the syringe with my right hand, and – it took me the longest of ten minutes to do this! – I held my breath, plunged the injection into my top left thigh, pressed the lever to inject the insulin, pulled it out, and breathed. Oh my gosh, what a feeling. Not just of pride, but relief. My audience, the two attending nurses, was as anxious and concerned as I. They clapped and congratulated me telling me what a good job I did, what a good girl I was! Phew! That is a great big deal when you are six year old!

With that accomplishment forever fastened in my knickers, I was off and running up to the "mess hall" for breakfast. Sometimes that hill seemed forever to climb due to a low blood glucose level or over exertion of exercise depending on time of day. Too many times I witnessed more than one child eating before the rest of us. That was due to an "insulin reaction," which requires food or a balanced sustenance quickened through liquid glucose for the insulin to act upon. The immediate use of "coke syrup" was available as well for such occasions. Thick and terribly sweet, I recall the nastiness of having to endure this treatment. It was necessary. An approximate twenty minutes would revive the child to her original personality.

Upon entering this two-room building, there was table after table of excitedly and happy talking children while breakfast scents of eggs, dry cereal, hot cereal, fresh fruit, milk and juice surrounded the children and councilors. The first area off to the left of the entrance was the kitchen. An oversized metal counter used for food serving was open to the diners. It took me a few minutes to locate my cabins' table and its members who were already seated along with our councilors. "Andy, we're over here!" exclaimed all of them in intervals. "Hurry up, we're hungry. Don't let it get cold!" They waited for me! I was flattered. Climbing over the picnic bench that was assigned to our cabin, I sat and had to wait again. With breakfast foods displayed on the picnic-styled tables along with a food-weighing scale, my senses drooled with anticipation, a food scale, of course, was purposely and distinctly used for each child's required caloric intake. Each entrée was separately matched to each of eighty-four campers, and oftentimes both of their diabetic councilors. It was up to the two councilors assigned to each cabin to weigh each child's food portion before themselves.

With that done, we all, the whole room, had to wait to say grace together. This occurred over each and every meal, every day. Respect was given.

During breakfast, councilors told us our daily schedules: activities for the day were discussed with their appropriate times; the required and intermittent snacks twice a day and where to get them; daily mail call; and whatever else to expect. Each camper and her cabin mates met again at lunch and dinner with the councilors reminding us of afternoon activities. There was a choice of swimming, badminton, volley ball, tennis, and basketball, hiking, making crafts, or writing letters home. Movement was constant with these activities scheduled by age group, ability and appropriateness. Learn, learn, learn.

Bright young adult faces belonging to adolescent campers, known as "CITs" (Councilors in Training) greeted each and every camper throughout the day, directing where a child should be as well as teaching many, like me, how to perform a certain activity. They were guardian angels! For instance, I didn't know how to play badminton until taught; I didn't know how to swim until taught; or how to row a boat or handle a canoe. It was the same with all the activities I participated in.

Unbeknownst to newcomers at the time, like me, we eventually became the soldiers of diabetes. Our examples were the older girls. They had already been living with this routine to assist in their own disease.

Another of many wonderful experiences was the every-evening-campfire. These occurred before bed or "lights out" as the counselors called it. We were encouraged to hold hands in a huge circle inclusive all campers, all councilors, most of the medical and administrative staffs. Singing out loud, *very* loud and together, constituted a main theme. Conversations about the days' occurrences took place with the expectations of what tomorrow would bring. Many, if not all, of the CIT's gave their learned reports of a days' event and updates of things to come such as a volleyball game or a hike to a certain area. It was practice in socialization with each other. Sometimes the boys in the Joslin Camp (named after Dr. Elliott P. Joslin) would participate in this affair.

We all learned to be crafty, creative, and imaginative human beings. It was our childhood. We learned to look forward to a productive life. We were, separately and together, continuously and eagerly encouraged toward progression, individually and socially.

Just the thought that possibilities were available was awesome! Unfathomable! Uncharted territories of the heart, mind, and soul!

One summer, stationed in the infirmary, was the familiar face of my doctor, my beloved Dr. Charles Graham. I couldn't believe it! He never mentioned a thing when I saw him last just a few weeks ago. After all, I had to see him before being able to come to camp in order to get all checked out properly with a healthy permission slip. I bet he wanted to surprise me. Well, he did! He was a delightfully humorous man with a southern accent, and had been the overseer of my disease for a few years already at this time. I remember being totally surprised and enthralled at his being there at CBC one summer. He was the doctor 'in charge.' But it wasn't just me he had to attend to. I was a bit jealous when I saw him speaking to another of the girls, or when he played on a volley team other than mine.

That particular summer, I was 12 years old. With his knowledge and guidance, my caloric intake was increased, allowing me to gain some weight and "fill out" more as I entered puberty.

I vividly recall the day that that summer session ended. My mother arrived to pick me up, my younger siblings in tow. As soon as she saw me in front of the "Lakeside Cabin" where I lived for those three weeks, she was startled at the weight I gained. I was happy to see her and my brother and two younger sisters. However, she was not happy to see me in this chubby state. The Sunday dress I had packed and was wearing for their arrival, a sheer, empire-waisted, white and brown number with brown polka dots, was a bit tight. I was embarrassed

After marching to the infirmary to get an explanation from Dr. Graham, whom she was surprised to see for herself, she settled down and concurred with his opinion. I needed more food to counteract the insulin and exercise I was getting. I was growing, developing into a young woman. Mom just had to face reality. Dr. Graham was the one to have repeatedly lead her to it. For a time, he was my spokesperson. He never knew it, but I always wished he was my father.

I was 13 when finally able to experience the tented area. This area was darker and cooler due to the canvassing overhang of the surrounding pine tree limbs. The smell - oh that luscious early morning wet pine smell - once again greeted me each day and remained throughout. So clean, so fresh.

Treated as an older camper, some of the rules changed, the daily schedules changed, responsibilities were aloft and implied. I felt this implication from being an older sister at home. No longer were pee pots carried for morning fasts. That would have been disastrous through a dark, damp wood at 7am. As a group of approximately eight teenage girls, it took at least fifteen minutes for all of us to make it out of the wood into the light at paths' end, across the asphalt road, through the dewy wet lawn near the mess hall, down the hill past the infirmary, only to arrive at the lavatory. Pajama clad, our pee pots awaited us in a neat and designated row in the lavatory. The routine was the same: pee in pot, bring to counter for testing, slosh through the morning slop left by the younger kids, wash hands, hike back up the hill for shots, and then cross the still-wet-crushed-to-mud-lawn to the mess hall. I quickly learned that wearing slippers was out of the question. Put on the sneakers as soon as you are awakened! Add the ingredient of languor to this daily process due to our ages. Teenagers, after all, do not move quickly.

Remaining in our pajamas through breakfast, as a team once again, we became listeners and watchers. But we were also watched – by young eyes – in our disarray. The little kids loved us and wanted to grow up, not necessarily to be like us with our "big girl privileges," but just to be able grow up with this disease. We were now supposed to be good examples.

For this experience, part of my personal packing gear included a bigger flashlight, extra batteries and a sleeping bag. I was cool, the envy of my siblings, at least. Specially purchased items without it being my birthday or Christmas were pretty rare in this family's budget!

Nearby, across the main entrance road and down about a quarter-of-a-mile, there was a small area resembling a chapel with approximately twenty wooden benches - two rows of ten benches each on each side of a wooden podium. With the sky as the roof, religious services were respectfully held here. After all, diversification without discrimination was the norm. Religious beliefs were respected and taken into account for the betterment of each person, be it child or adult. In later years, and due to the deterioration and vandalism of this chapel, services were held in the original barn on the property.

The CBC pond is a man-made pond in close proximity to this first "summer home" ("Squirrel's Nest") where my young colleagues and I learned to swim. First having to hold your breath, placing one's face in the water and blowing bubbles thereafter lead to many years of safe exercise in any body of water. We were 5 and 6 years old. As natural as natural can be, dog paddling was accomplished. At the end of the semester, each of us earned and received a "patch" for this, our proud accomplishment. We diabetics could swim! Other patches of accomplishment were also handed out, as deserved, for volley ball, tennis, badminton, track, archery, basketball, canoeing, row boating, sailing, etc. Through the years, I received one or two of each patch, delighted with myself to be able to participate in such activities.

Although the pond was full of leeches, they didn't stop any campers or their counselors from swimming. Hot and heavily humid summer days necessitated a swimming hole, any swimming hole!

I vividly recall screams from one youngster to another about a leech being on their body. Counselors in close proximity would always rush with a book of matches to burn off the sucker! Ah, memories. This happened to the adults as well, but the drama wasn't as peaked. I've witnessed, time and time again, another counselor purposely scoping the body of another counselor with matches in hand. Many times those matches were put to good use.

But the pond was also used for canoe and row–boat lessons. This was the first time I was ever in either type of boat. I found rowing to be more difficult than paddling. However, my adventurous spirit would never hesitate to get into either vehicle, especially once I learned how to swim. Such exercise was encouraged, usually after breakfast, with a paddle or row on the outer right edges of the pond, under the walking bridge, and back again via the other side. Gosh, that was the best! Both activities I have continued into my adult life.

During the closing engagements of many of my three-week stays, one counselor volunteered to swim the length of the pond with a lit torch in her hand. This task was wonderfully and amazingly accomplished. And, as always, afterwards she was physically scanned for the "attack of the leeches." Such a feat encouraged me to think that "I could do that!" It was greatly encouraging.

With the volleyball net conveniently located across from our cabin, my first introduction to this sport began. I recall not being the strongest of players, but I put my heart into it. Oftentimes, tournaments and "Olympics" were held upon occasion as an exciting summer afternoon event. Personally, this was my first introduction to competition of any sort. Most often, one cabin competed against another. This initially formed a team spirit and practice before children from other camps were bused to ours, or vice versa, for such events. When we CBC campers traveled, coolers of supplies were in tow holding food and medicine. It was more fun to watch the counselors compete against each other as each camper routed for her cabin captain.

For example, one such Olympic memory involved my running track when I was about 11 years old. Through constant encouragement and practice, I ran the 100-yard dash in 14.7 seconds. That accomplishment was my entrance into that physical race. However, I did not win. Another girl from another camp who was larger and stronger than I won that race.

Further introductions into how to build a fire with rocks and twigs, canoeing, sailing, leather and beaded craft making, playing tennis, basketball, softball, and so on were fashioned for each age group.

Once getting home, I always brought my mother a present I had made in the "Craft Cabin."

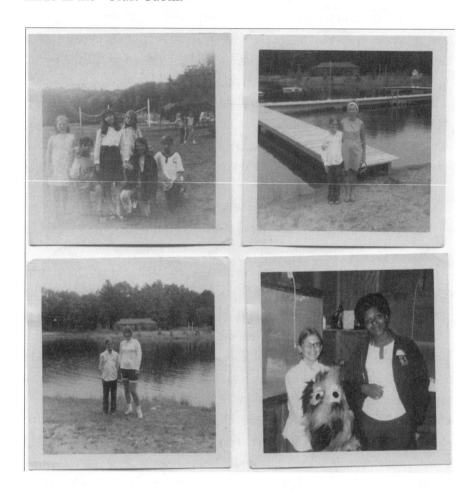

Special outings, always on a Sunday, were spent at Dr. Elliot P. Joslin's home in North Oxford, Massachusetts. His brief autobiography follows:

"Elliott Proctor Joslin, M.D. *(6 June 1869 - 28 January 1962) was the first doctor in the United States to specialize in diabetes and was the founder of today's Joslin Diabetes Center. He was the first to advocate for teaching patients to care for their own diabetes, an approach now commonly referred to as "DSME" or Diabetes Self-Management Education. He is also a recognized pioneer in glucose* *management, identifying that tight glucose control leads to fewer and less extreme complications.*

"He was born in 1869 in Oxford, Massachusetts and educated at Leicester Academy, Yale College and Harvard Medical School.

"Joslin first became interested in diabetes while attending Yale, when his aunt was diagnosed with the disease. At the time, diabetes was considered an obscure disease, with no cure and little hope. He made diabetes his focus while attending Harvard Medical School, winning the Boylston Society prize for work later published as the book The Pathology of Diabetes Mellitus.

"His postgraduate training was at Massachusetts General Hospital, and he also studied with leading researchers in metabolism from Germany and Austria before starting a private medical practice in Boston's Back Bay in 1898.

"In 1908, in conjunction with physiologist Francis G. Benedict, Joslin carried out extensive metabolic balance studies examining fasting and feeding in patients with varying severities of diabetes. His findings would help to validate the observations of Frederick Madison Allen regarding the benefit of carbohydrate- and calorie-restricted diets. The patients were admitted to units at New England Deaconess Hospital, helping to initiate a program to help train nurses to supervise the rigorous diet program.

"Joslin included the findings from 1,000 of his own cases in his 1916 monograph The Treatment of Diabetes Mellitus. Here he noted a 20 percent decrease in the mortality of patients after instituting a program of diet and exercise. This physician's handbook had 10 more editions in his lifetime and established Dr. Joslin as a world leader in diabetes. "Two years later, Dr. Joslin wrote Diabetic Manual — for the Doctor and Patient detailing what patients could do to take control of their disease. This was the first diabetes patient

handbook and became a best seller. There have been 14 editions of this pioneering patient handbook, and a version is still published today by the Joslin Diabetes Center under the title The Joslin Guide to Diabetes.

"When insulin became available as therapy in 1922, Joslin's corps of nurses became the forerunners of certified diabetes educators, providing instruction in diet, exercise, foot care and insulin dosing, and established camps for children with diabetes throughout New England.

"Dr. Joslin always adopted a multi-disciplinary approach, working with nurses in education, surgeons and podiatrists for limb salvage and foot care, pathologists for descriptions of complications and obstetricians for assessment of fetal risk in diabetic pregnancy. The first hospital blood glucose monitoring system for pre-meal testing was developed under his direction in 1940, and was the forerunner of modern home-monitoring systems.

"Dr. Joslin was also the first to name diabetes as a serious public health issue. Just after WWII, he expressed concern to the Surgeon General of the U.S. Public Health Service that diabetes was an epidemic and challenged the government to do a study in the town of his birthplace, Oxford, Massachusetts. The study was started in 1946 and carried out over the next 20 years. The results would later confirm Joslin's fear that the incidence of diabetes in the United States was approaching epidemic proportions. He has been named as being, along with Frederick Madison Allen, one of the two leading diabetologists from the period between 1910 and 1920.

"In 1952, Joslin's group practice became officially known as the Joslin Clinic. In 1956, the office was moved to its current location at One Joslin Place in Boston. Joslin Clinic was the world's first diabetes care facility and today maintains its place as the largest diabetes clinic in the world.

Dr. Joslin was adamant in his position that good glucose control, achieved through a restricted carbohydrate diet, exercise, and frequent testing and insulin adjustment, would prevent complications. This was debated for decades by other endocrinologists and scientists, and the American Diabetes Association was divided on this subject from its inception. Joslin's approach was not validated until 30 years after his death, when in 1993, a 10-year study, "The Diabetes Control and Complications Trial Report" was published in the prestigious New England Journal of Medicine. "This study demonstrated that the onset of diabetes complications was delayed by tight glucose control, something Joslin had argued decades prior.

"Dr. Joslin died in his sleep on 29 January 1962 in Brookline, Massachusetts."
(Retrieved from: http://en.wikipedia.org/wiki/Elliott_P._Joslin.)

There were occasions during my camping sessions when all campers and most of the staff were bused to Dr. Joslin's spacious family farm estate in North Oxford. The estate entrance itself was as delightful as a fairy tale. The private dirt roadway leading to the spacious home was neatly lined with tree after tree, providing a coolly shaded welcome on the hot Sunday afternoons that I was there. We children cajoled him and his wife and staff with camp songs, walked the vast and beauteous grounds, visited with the geese, pigs, cows, horses and whatever else were available. The 3:00 afternoon snack of watermelon slices were graciously passed all around. I had never seen so many watermelons in my life since those days and probably never will. It is a tremendously happy memory!

I further recall my very first summer visiting the farm, impressionistic and naïve as I was. I was chided into milking a cow. Having yielded to my fellow campers' teasing remarks, I was gently guided by a ranch-hand to sit upon a small wooden stool aside a cow. He softly explained and showed me at the same time how to gently and cautiously grab a nipple on the cow's udder and squeeze. My audience was silenced, enthralled that I could do this.

At one point, I squeezed too hard, causing the cow to shift her weight. This, in turn, caused me to squirt milk in my face. Laughter ensued by me and my audience. However, "Mrs. Cow" so-called turned her big head towards me, looked at me, and wagged her tail in my face, wiping away the spilt milk. I couldn't believe it! I was in awe along with all the other kids who were now screaming amid laughter to "Let me! Let me!" Well, that was that for the farm hand. No other child that day was allowed to milk Mrs. Cow.

Chapter 6
Eyeballs, gateways to the rest of you.

As a child, the majority of my time was spent at home and school, of course, with the tri-monthly doctor visits to include an ophthalmologist and optician. Due to the infamous diabetes complication of retinopathy, this visit remains a dire and yearly necessity.

> **"Diabetic retinopathy:** *A common complication of Diabetes affecting the blood vessels in the retina (the thin light-sensitive membrane that covers the back of the eye). If untreated, it may lead to blindness. If diagnosed and treated promptly, blindness is usually preventable."* **(www.medscape.com.)**

Mr. Lewandowski was the doctor of choice, our family eye doctor/optometrist. His office was conveniently located down the hill from school and appointments were conveniently made after school. Usually one or two of my siblings were seen at the same time. Mom would meet us there after her work shift, get the doctors' report, and take us all home.

A very kind, gentle, and realistic man, Dr. Lewandowski was more than thorough with his examinations. My being diagnosed with nearsightedness at the age of seven gave cause to my having to wear glasses.

Once this first pair of glasses was fitted properly, I tried them out and was sternly told that I would be wearing them every day. My school chums didn't seem surprised or aghast when I arrived at school the next morning. I remember being surprised at their non-surprise! I still wonder if they were lectured before hand by our teacher as to not make fun of me. Yes, in forthcoming years the term "four eyes" was used to get my attention in an insulting manner. Having to wear glasses also meant that I no longer had to sit in front of the class. I did not – and do not – like to sit up front anywhere.

During these continual, yearly visits, I was introduced to the word "retinopathy." Because it is a noun denoting negative consequences, it's a bad word for me. Retinopathy is one of many possible complication of diabetes that leads to blindness. *All* the complications – the sicknesses - are terribly horrible. And there are consequences for *everything* – everything you do and don't do. If a person has retinopathy, s/he also has kidney failure. I quickly learned the meaning of the phrase "your eyes are a reflection of your soul." To me this means that whatever can be seen in the structure of an eyeball, especially through yearly dilating examinations, literally displays other negative possibilities, future encumbrances. Therefore, I have been reminded once again to take care of myself, to listen to the doctors, and that I am ultimately in control of my person.

The following pages' photograph of my eyeballs was taken in May, 2003. I am proud of this photograph and wish to share it with you. Keep in mind that that year I was diabetic for forty-four years. Many of the last ten years now I have tolerated "floaters," a sign of retinopathy. Seen as small black dots obscuring my vision, they represent broken blood vessels in the eyes. Not good. Broken blood vessels inhibit light to shine into the retina, causing distortion and blindness. I don't like the floaters. Not only are they more bothersome at times than others, but they scare me concerning the possibility of blindness. These "black dots" first appeared to me while viewing a computer monitor at work. The office was bright and I believed there were bugs flying around me. I complained that the packs of newly ordered computer paper must have bugs in them. As these "tiny bugs" insisted on flying in my face, I continued to swat at them. Other office personnel came to see what I was blaring about and they could see nothing. "It's your imagination," I was told and joked at. Okay, I conceded, after being totally embarrassed.

This specific circumstance leads me to the optometrist's office who leads me to the ophthalmologist's office who bravely told me I had "floaters" with a full explanation. Twice-yearly visits to an ophthalmologist are necessitated at this stage of my life. Sure, an ophthalmologists' examination is uncomfortable and it hurts, but it has to be done. Having my eyes dilated at these visits allows the doctor to view the back of my eyeball. It feels like he is viewing the back of my brain! With an extremely bright light strapped to his forehead, I am told to move an eye up, down, left, and right. Viewed from all angles, a prognosis is told me and written in my record for all time.

Driving home is a slow chore. Sensitivity to light, daylight or artificial, is *extremely* uncomfortable. Wearing two pairs of sunglasses, one atop the other, has allowed me to drive. After having done this for many years, I no longer ask for someone to pick me up, causing him or her to have to take time off from work. I try to keep it simple.

My recovery period has been twenty-four hours after this process: my eyes no longer hurt from being stretched, the headache disappears, and my vision normalizes.

I never did live down "the swatting action" and continue to chuckle when a former colleague would imitate my actions. I continue to laugh out loud at the memory!

Furthermore, having researched this "spotty" predicament, I came up with the action of exercising my eyeballs. Yes, moving them from side-to-side at the top of my head and then at the bottom. This enables oxygen to get to the eye balls. That's what exercise is all about – oxygen for blood circulation. This action helps a little bit, but doesn't make the dots go away.

Stove-top-popcorn was prepared and presented to us as we gathered around the television. I was allowed a six-ounce cup of it for my evening snack. Well, I wanted more. Marcy was seriously watching me, policing me once again, and knowing what I was going to do. I think I may have quickly grabbed that handful of popcorn to taunt her, to challenge her. As my older sister, implications of her life were foresworn to watch over me. Well, she did her job!

Before I knew it, Marcy was screaming "Mom, Andrea's eating more popcorn." Well, we all froze. We knew I was in trouble. Mom came immediately, pounding down the cellar stairs, grabbed my arm, and practically dragged me back up those stairs. It was awful!

RETINAL CONSULTANTS
MEDICAL GROUP

Andrea Buckroth
Diagnosis:

11/6/2006
Photographer: MCA

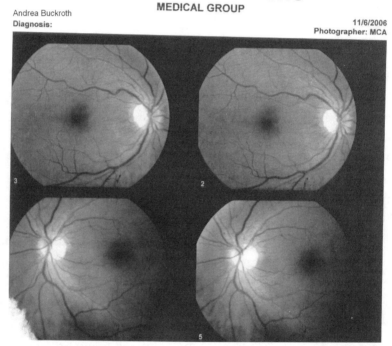

Amidst her babbling anger and my crying, my mother managed to tie a scarf around my head to purposely cover my eyes. "This is what it's like to be blind," she screamed. "Do you like that? Is this what you want?! You walk around like that. Go ahead, walk, see if you can. Walk up and down the hall. Go. *Now*!"

I did. I cried through that scarf. I was scared. I was humiliated.

Impressionable, I got the point.

I cried so hard that the scarf was so wet I could have squeezed out my tears. I was afraid. I don't know if I was more afraid of my mother or this fact of this disease!

Tough love, that's what that was.

I don't remember much else of that night. The remembrance makes me tired. My dislike of Marcy being a tattle-tail was born that night.

As an older camper aged 13 and 14, my first introduction to boys as social members of society took place at weekend dances. Sure, I have a brother, be it a younger brother, and there were always boys at school, but this was so totally different! My self-consciousness arose, however, due to having to wear glasses. Made fun of with the typical phrase of being called "four eyes," I shut myself out and away from boys. I soon felt I was unliked and unwanted because I wore glasses. Stigmatized, the only thing I could do was to accept this.

The Joslin Diabetes Center's boys' camp, founded by Dr. Elliot Joslin, was three miles away. Often, an exercise routine from CBC to the Joslin Camp involved a 3-mile hike to their part of the woods or vice versa for a social event. Yellow buses would take us back after such events.

During these youthful summers, lifelong friendships, especially memories, endure to this day. Outside of camp, many of us became pen-pals, exchanging letters that continued into adulthood. Faces with names and personalities that shared youthful adventures in early girlhood such as that belonging to Lisa K., Diane C., Maxine A., Allison, Kathy M., Debbie C., "New York" Buffie, Cathy C., my sisters Gina and Judy, Debbie L., Trisha, Mary Lou, Patti K., and too many more to mention are displayed in the following photographs. You may recognize faces in the adjacent pictures. Many of these youngsters have since passed away due to diabetes complications. Upon the recent 2008 passing of Cathy C., I pulled out some thirty-year-old photographs with her and I photographed side-by-side as campers, as friends. It's awful to realize that I may be the only one alive among these pictures.

The whole aspect of CBC was to train all these children into adulthood toward happy and fulfilling lives. With all this training and personal attention, I often thought that I was brainwashed. I had to be. It was a necessity. The constant drilling of "insulin, diet and exercise" *had* to be a life routine. It is. I now realize that this disease has been a blessing. Yes, I wrote that right: a blessing. I've been purposely made and learned to eat a proper human diet, I learned self-disciple, self-respect, and limitations of others as well as myself. I have learned to pray hard, for myself and others, asking my Holy Guardian Angels, Messengers of God, to bring *my* messages, my requests for health, happiness, and a cure to God Almighty. I believe. Diabetes has insisted that I not become an alcoholic or a drug addict. It has kept me safe and wholesome. I do not want to be a statistic.

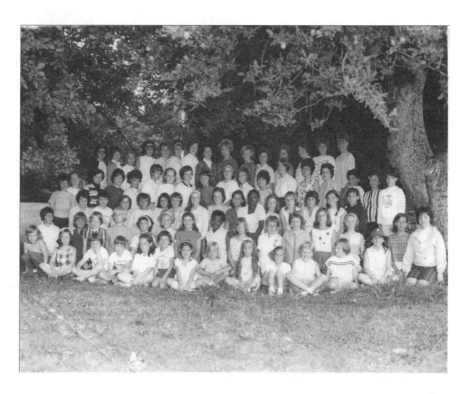

Yes, there were a few summers at CBC when my eye glasses were broken through no fault of my own. They always broke at the nose piece, right in half, where they could be taped together and I could continue wearing them until I got home, visited Dr. Lewandowski's office and repairs were made. What a geek! Trying to be ever-so-careful, I tucked them under my bunk pillow before falling asleep. That was really the only convenient and easy place to put them for quick morning access. Heck, I couldn't see without them. Vanity was not an issue for me, not at camp, so the tape was no big deal.

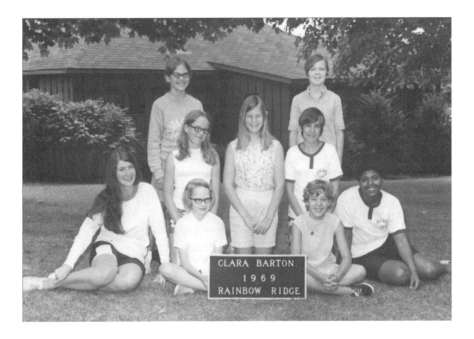

Wearing what eventually amounted to coke-bottle glasses continued until I was approximately twenty-six years old, I was finally able to replace them with contact lenses. A vain decision, my glasses were like wearing actual "coke-bottles," getting thicker, heavier, and uglier each year. I put off this wearing of contacts for so long, being frightened, not knowing if this choice would worsen my diabetic eyes. Well, the decision became a good one. Contacts actually allow more oxygen to the eyes and displayed my pair of gorgeously large, dark browns that I didn't know I had.

Interestingly enough, a "Pennsylvania based company called Sentek Group has come up with a new, non-invasive way of monitoring diabetes that doesn't require any pricey machinery. Called the 'Glucoview,' the noninvasive monitoring device is a disposable contact lens that is placed on the eye and changes color according to glucose levels in tear fluid. A patient matches the lens hue to a calibrated color wheel inside a compact mirror with each shade corresponding to a glucose level." (***Diabetes Interview,* D. Trecroci © 2001.**)

Although I came across this article many years after my introduction to wearing contacts, I couldn't help but wonder how cool would that be. Imagine sitting in a restaurant for dinner, and a persons' eye color begins to change, first by fluctuations of shading then completely something different, like orange! Ooh, creepy! This inventive idea reminds me of those Clinitest tablets I used as a child. The memories are not that good. In fact, I wouldn't want anyone to know I was actively messing up while having a beer or sneaking a chocolate chip cookie. Those and so many other food items with instances (e.g., becoming sick, being angry, etc.) would literally be displayed through my eye color. Nah. By wearing contact lenses, I wanted to be able to see without the impediments of glasses and further display my own dream of having beauty and poise!

"Dreams are illustrations…from the book your soul is writing about you."
~ Marsha Norman ~

Once school ended around June 10th of each year, my sisters, brother and I, were *strictly* disciplined on taking care of each other. Mom *had* to work. This not only included what chores were to be performed each day by each child, but what was to be prepared for lunch and supper, and to call Mrs. M., our neighbor, if there was an emergency. I believe this is when I learned to let others know my secret, that I was a diabetic. Such a fact was diminished as I got older what with higher education and career building.

You see, Mrs. M. was a nurse and mother of the four neighborhood children that we played with on a daily basis. They lived four houses away. She was also a sister-in-law to my late Uncle John, mom's oldest brother.

Susan, Mrs. M's oldest child and between Marcy and my ages, always came over to keep us company, see what was up and the like. We were not allowed to leave the yard. I was a curiosity to Susan. Having to eat mid-morning and mid-afternoon snacks seemed to intrigue her. One time, as I was munching on a graham cracker, she wanted a piece. Not being able to share my allotment, so to speak, I went in the house to get a cracker for her. Well, she didn't want her own. She wanted to share mine. She went home upset, not understanding what I earnestly tried to tell her. Maybe she didn't believe me. Whatever. Her mom more than likely discussed my dietary needs with Susan that afternoon. We resumed our friendship the next day.

Daily listening to radio station WORC with host Jeff Starr at the time, we sang our favorite songs and grew together. Mud pies were baked in the backyard sun; clubhouses were built from stray wood that was found; toy car highways were constructed in the dirt; dolls were dressed, walked, bathed, and re-dressed. Kid stuff. The worse to happen on any summer day to my recollection was when either one of my siblings being angry at another, slammed the screen door, causing it to break. There was a time that we got our dog all riled up and excited that he jumped through the glass of that same door, unscathed. That was scary. What was even scarier was having to explain to mom how and why this happened – again!

Saturday walks to the neighborhood Billings Square Library on Hamilton Street were enjoyable. My siblings and I greatly enjoyed reading then as now. I also like to call myself "a well-read" person. The only books I never finished were *The Rise and Fall of the Third Riech* by William Shirer and *The Iliad* by Homer translated by W.

H. D. Rouse. The first I stopped at page 909 of 1143 where a book mark remains to this day. The second holds a book mark at page 92 of 297. I just can't force myself to read them as yet. However, I consider these readings as tasks that will be overcome. There is hope as with everything in this life!

To continue, the book check-out allowance at the library was six books per child. I took this limit and walked them home two miles. Occasionally I'd help a sister with her load as well, or vice versa.

These excursions gave mom a break and we kids were allowed to visit the ice cream parlor on the walk home. It was known as "Smithfield's Ice Cream Parlor." There were two positives with these excursions: Marcy had instructions, *and* money, on what we could each get. My ice cream was always a plain cone with one scoop of a fruit-based ice cream – banana, blackberry, or strawberry – especially with big, fat fruit pieces in it. Chunks of fruit are always tastier, more daring. This concept has continued throughout my life. There is a "guilt-free" value of ordering a fruit-based ice cream as opposed to ever-popular chocolate, caramel, or other flavors with chunks of candy. I didn't bother with vanilla. It was too boring. But that treat was well-deserved as well as well-planned. There was no sugar-free ice cream in those days! My brother and sisters always chose the chunky-chocolate-with-nut types of ice creams. Nuts and chunks did not matter to me. I was happy that we were all happy together after such a delightful treat!

Chapter 7
Beach-Life-Lessons

Out of school for the summer, Misquamicut Beach in Westerly, Rhode Island, was a monthly excursion. I don't recall how mom found out about this particular piece of the Atlantic Ocean, but we kids didn't care. We had a blast! Each Saturday trip turned out to be an adventurous family excursion. They were wonderfully and habitually full of memorable summer family activities. A few trips were made before I was packed off to summer camp and another trip or two was made after my return.

You must realize that the prospect of any adventure in my immediate horizon with my brother and sisters involved minute preparations to detail. Visited two or three times during any summer, such preparations to detail were well planned and rehearsed. With five children in a green station wagon, my mother was the coordinating and detailed leader. We kids were her assistants, especially my older sister and I. I swear that this is how I learned to be so organized as a multi-tasker.

When mom said "we're going to Misquamicut on Saturday" we knew what had to be done; there was no problem! For instance, having to bring the large metal cooler upstairs from its storage spot in the basement and cleaning it out and dusting it off; packing towels and a full change of clothes for everyone; making sure all our bathing suits still fit and needed repairs, replacements, or not. Chucky's swim trunks never seemed to need replacing. It was most likely Marcy and/or Judy that needed new suits. I got Marcy's hand-me-down from the summer before and Gina got mine. Being so young, we didn't care about stylin.' Heck, we were going to Misquamicut!

The clothes preparing was easy. It was the food preparation that took more time and detail. Eggs were boiled, chicken wings broiled, carrots, celery, cucumbers washed and sliced; cheese and sandwich meat with bread were packed after being freshly purchased from the deli. Gosh, how we all loved fresh deli-sandwich meats! Two tightly-as-possible lidded plastic containers – one with sweetened Kool-Aid for the non-diabetics, one with plain water and another with orange juice - were packed amid ice cubes from the freezer's metal ice cube trays. Fresh fruits were included. Usually bringing a whole watermelon was sufficient for the six of us. Dry goods included cups, napkins, a knife for the watermelon, salt and pepper shakers, and, of course, toys (e. g., shovels with buckets, a beach ball that was usually destroyed, plastic trucks and cars, a Frisbee, maybe a badminton set). Mom had her coffee thermos. It was a regular picnic.

Before our Babci's passed away, she did have an occasion to venture with us to this beach, bringing her best friend, Pañi Koparcz. It was great fun to watch these old women conquering the ocean waves! Hardy, strong and hefty women they dove right in, certain to secure their bathing caps, whooping, hollering, and out of breath once they were done. There was absolutely no defeating their joyful spirits. It was a hilariously joyful sight to see, especially as they happily and freely hallooed in Polish! Before plunging into the roily Atlantic Ocean, these women would bless themselves, making the sign of the cross on their foreheads and chests. I respected that action and have adopted it throughout my life. After all, we were all Catholics here. I recall being astounded at their enthusiasm and excitement. With mom, we watched them, awestruck, staring, as they fearlessly dove into the ocean time and time again. I learned from their example. Vanity was non-existent.

On another specific occasion at this beach, I recall standing ashore near our picnic spot in the hot sand, looking into the crowd, watching people and the ocean. Gina ran past me, toward mother, screaming "Andrea's dancing! Andrea's dancing." I heard Gina loud and clear. My left leg, thigh to ankle was shaking as if it was dancing by itself. I didn't feel a thing as I stood there, watching and witnessing the active scenery. "Andrea, sit. Andrea, sit," mother commanded as she flew up behind me, cup of orange juice in hand. "Sit on the blanket. Can't you feel what's happening?!" she exclaimed. No, I did not feel a thing and was oblivious to my shaking. I really didn't know what the excitement was all about. Drinking the juice, doused with I don't know how many packets of sugar, I slowly stopped shaking and leveled off to normalcy. Quickly followed with lunch, my brother and sisters watched me in a stupor. Anxious and nervous, it took more than a few minutes for them to gain composure enough to indulge in their own sandwiches. Gina saved me – again.

A short time later, Marcy took me aside at the ocean's edge and confronted me about what happened, wanting to know why and how I couldn't sense or feel what took place. She was upset. I couldn't answer her. We were all upset. My siblings not only saw this open demonstration of a convulsive activity, they felt it along with me, especially the embarrassment. Onlookers, wondering what the hullabaloo was all about with 'those kids,' didn't know our secret. It was that day, at the approximate age of eleven that I vowed to myself to learn my body signals. I knew how to combat them with the ever-present orange juice. I now desperately needed to pay attention to my body's warning signs. I didn't want to put any of us through such a fiasco ever again! I *had* to learn!

Year after year in those early summer times when all of us kids were done with school, when mom got her vacation time, we, as a young family, spent quality time at Misquamicut Beach. Together we became extremely familiar with its neighborhoods and community. After a few years of driving back and forth, mom was able to afford to rent us a cottage. We stayed on Ginger Lane in a cabin called Ginger. Gosh, that was so much easier with five kids and all the stuff each of us wanted to bring, and pack, into the beloved station wagon.

Wow! This was a *big* deal! We were going to stay at Misquamicut or the *whole* week!

Chucky and Gina were now old enough to help Marcy and I pack everything but the kitchen sink and separately organize everybody's individual stuff. Overwhelmed with excitement, this job was done without a complaint, or a bicker or a whine. We kids worked well together when we wanted to.

With the station wagon packed to the brim, our course was set for our beloved Westerly, Rhode Island, once again. Marcy always got to sit in the passenger-side front seat with mom and Judy in between. As the co-pilot, Marcy had to watch for the highway signs to make sure we were going in the right direction. Mom had a tendency to get lost by taking the wrong right turn, or was it the left? As soon as Marcy would yell out "Route 145," it was verified by the backseat echoers. One particular summer when Marcy had just received her driving permit, she was ever so studious and attentive to road signs and safety precautions. My seat was always behind mom. It seemed I was purposely placed there so that she could see and watch me through the rear-view mirror. At this age, I was finally able to foretell and declare an insulin reaction, bet mom was always on the alert, precautious. You know, "an ounce of prevention is worth a pound of cure." Actually, I think mom watched me in that mirror to make sure I was watching the other two: Gina sitting next to me and Chucky at the door. Those were our permanent family car-sitting arrangements.

Arriving at the cabin on Ginger Lane at mid-morning, unpacking was heeded to immediately and with anxious excitement. We wanted to get to the beach! Not possible until things were settled in the cottage. Not a problem. Once again, we worked well together.

I received my first boy-kiss on the evening sands of Misquamicut Beach. I do not remember his name but I do remember my top lip getting caught in his braces. How embarrassing! We were 14 years old.

Adventures were numerous, always finding something new and exciting from the historical cemetery dating back to 1868 or Point Judith, Watch Hill, an Indian Museum or the Andrea Hotel for New

England lobsters. The experiences were never ending. The ride home was always topped off with a picnic supper at "the well." This was a small park-type area, more of a secluded rest stop for weary travelers such as us. Picnic tables inhabited by black ants and large pine trees of varying heights provided a cool shady spot at the end of our day. It was quiet and private, as if no one knew about it. The well's water pumping handle never worked, but it was fun *to try* and make it work. Maybe it needed a child's magic. Nevertheless, the area was worth a timely adventure. Whatever leftovers were finished up, allowing most of us, myself included, to snooze on the ride to *Janet's Ice Cream Parlor* further down the road closer to home. That was time for dessert! Oftentimes, mom allowed me and my diet to "cheat" just a bit and order one scoop of a chunky ice cream mixture as opposed to my typical fruit based flavors. Ah, those trips were exhausting from sheer delight! Each of us, in turn, expressed a delightful dream of hoping to live in that area 'when we grew up.'

Feet. Feet care with diabetics is so vitally important if only because of poorer circulation in the lower extremities of the human body. Think about it. Basically, cuts, bruises, blisters, scratches, bug bites, corns, calluses, in-grown toenails, whatever harm may come to a diabetics' foot or feet has to be tended to immediately. It really is important to a non-diabetic as well. At the sake of repeating myself, circulation is poorer, slower, in the human body's lower extremities causing not only a slower healing process, but a larger chance of infection. Diabetics do not do well with infections anywhere on or in their bodies, but it has always been implied to me that any abrasion below the knee could become catastrophic.

With this in mind, going bare foot was practically a crime for me as a child. Wearing open toed/heeled sandals was no better. There were and have been too many times while wearing an open toe sandal or high-heel, some bit of something – a pebble, a splinter – got stuck in my foot or toe. For instance, after walking around with what I thought was a wart on the bottom of my left foot for two years, I finally saw a doctor. He removed a pebble. Can you imagine? There was a pebble imbedded in the skin of my foot! Amazing! The doctor was amazed as he held the pebbled in the air between the tweezers he used to remove it. I did receive a lecture, however. No, no drama. As long as I took care of that small incision – which I did - it healed wonderfully. Blessed again!

Feet protection at all times was and is the order of every day.

"Where are your slippers?" my mother would yell.

"Under my bed," I would say, knowing the response beforehand.

"Why aren't they on your feet?" she would quiz.

"I don't know," was my sheepish reply.

"Get them on!"

"Yes ma'am," I'd say and hop right to it, scrambling for my slippers or whatever footwear was available.

Summers were the worse time for having to wear shoes. They were just too bulky. *"Keds"* were popular and probably the only 'sneakers' back in my childhood and they were not popular. It was stereotypical that poor people wore canvas-on-rubber shoes. They were cheap. I'm talking $0.50 (fifty cents) a pair back then! Well, we had them. On our strict family budget with five children, $5.00 to cover ten feet for a summer was a deal!

Wearing shoes at the beach is just not cool. With this fact in mind, we always laid our blankets close to the shore for easy access in and out of the water. It just so happened on one of these excursions I happened to find a broken glass bottle with the bottom of my left heel. One of my siblings screamed as my foot bled. Limping away from the stinging, salt water, I plopped onto the beach blanket, examining this insult to my conscious innocence. After my mother examined the slice, she hailed a life guard who, with his first aid kit at hand, wiped out the cut and wrapped it in gauze. The rest of the day was spent on the blanket, watching my siblings play in the water. What a drag! Lesson learned.

To this day, I have kept a pair of slippers or slip-on sandals at each doorway to my home. There is a fact that never ceases to amaze me: when I am bare foot, inside or outside, my feet will find that missing piece of glass in the carpet, the sliver from the wood pile, the common pin, the dropped thumb-tack, or the rose thorn from the garden roses that were brought in the night before. Honest to goodness! Cover those feet! Avoid infection!

Chapter 8
Sugar-free, that's me!

One of the first sugar-free goodies I distinctly recall was something called *"fizzies."* I don't even know where my mother found and purchased them. I didn't care. They were pretty cool, creative and innovative-wise.

Comparable to the present day antacid item known as "Alka-Seltzer," fizzies could be dropped into a glass of water where one would fizz and be drunk. Available in a variety of flavors, orange was my favorite. I would also eat them whole, letting one flavor or the other fizz in my mouth. The root-beer flavored fizzie was also tasty. They made my tongue turn color, which was even cooler! Eating them that way caused my mouth to burn and become sore. I didn't care. Fizzies were for *me!* Occasionally I would allow my brother and sisters to experience a fizzie or two, but I never let my supply get too low. The neighbor kids were in awe and wanted to try them but they did not like them. I was already adapted to that sugar-free taste, the bitter twinge that is left in your mouth after eating or drinking something that is sugar-free. Fizzies are no longer available on a grand marketing scale, but I have been able to locate them at a small and private retailer.

Sugar-free chewing gum was introduced to me while at camp. Tasteless as this was, it was sheer joy that such a thing existed. However, it was like chewing on a tasteless piece of rubber and hardened quickly.

The introduction of a sugar-free soda, "TAB," was absolutely delightful. The following is a brief history of this product:

"**TaB** was Coca-Cola Company's first sugar-free drink, introduced in 1963. Its name was a play on the notion of people keeping "tabs" on their weight.

Although sales of **TaB** were surpassed by the introduction of diet Coke®, the brand still has fiercely loyal fans that have been known to travel hundreds of miles to find their favorite drink." **(http://www@lundy.org.)**

The availability of this delight was a splurge in my mother's budget. Although I was the only one to drink it in our household if only because my siblings didn't have an acquired taste for anything "sugar-free," mom found something else for them to enjoy.

Not far from our house was a small manufacturing plant on Millbury Street. Soda was made here, regular and sugar-free. I don't know how our mother ever found this place, but cases of soda were purchased for all of us in imaginative colorful flavors that included chocolate, raspberry, and lemon-lime. It was absolutely delightful! My mother was just plain ingenious at locating, or "hearing about" (networking) many items – be it people, places or things. She was always ahead of her time, quite trendy. Her findings were fun for all of us. If one was happy, we all were happy!

With all this soda and its colorful flavors, introduction of ice cream sodas was a great treat, always conscious of *how much* ice cream I was allowed.

At approximately the same time, another sugar-free soda product made its way into our household. Although not as appreciated as "TAB," mom bought this new "Fresca" for me and then helped me drink it. Thank goodness!

"Fresca is a brand of citrus soft drink made by the Coca-Cola Company. First introduced in the United States in 1963, the drink is now sold throughout the world. It is a rarity in Coke products, in that it does not have a Pepsi equivalent.

"Since its inception, Fresca has been marketed in the United States as a calorie-free, grapefruit-flavored soft drink, ostensibly catering to discriminating adult tastes. In 1985, the drink was given its one major ingredient change, in that it was now being sweetened with aspartame." **(http://www.en.wikipedia.org.)**

Due to my convulsive episodes, explained on page 110, and having to have orange juice physically induced down my throat, the citrusy taste of Fresca was of no interest.

There was another soda drink, called *Moxie* that also came in sugar-free and regular tastes. To me, it had a root beer taste with great bitters. I didn't like it, but consumed it to make others happy. My mother and her friends who occasionally visited us seemed to like it fine. Therefore, I considered it to be a fashionably *adult* drink. I wanted to be an adult as all children do, so I partook in it. However, I think that mom and her friends drank it to make me more comfortable with the limited sugar-free marketed items. It was a kindness that helped me feel that I belonged, that I could be socially acceptable. Moxie was available and usually purchased specifically for me because there was nothing else and people just wanted to be nice. However, I never liked it, with or without ice cream! I believe it had an *acquired* taste.

Another product I recall trying with my mother's encouragement was tiny white sweetening flavor tablets. A small clear glass jar contained perhaps 100 of these pills. To sweeten something such as a cup of tea, I would place one or two of these pills between two teaspoons and crush it, letting the powder swirl into the beverage. Two crushed pills were more than enough due to a bitter after taste.

And then the pink-envelope sweetener came along, then the blue, then the yellow. Using any of these products for many, many years, my cousin, Katrina brought the fact of "aspartame" to my attention. She was seriously distraught that I used such sweeteners and adamantly told me not to use them anymore. "That stuff is in everything sugar-free. It causes cancer. It causes brain tumors! It's in those diet sodas you drink and every other sugar-free product you eat. Get off of that stuff. Don't use it. Don't use anything!" The year was 1988 or 1989.

Gosh, she really made me think. She scared me into thinking about this! And I cut down my use drastically, getting back to going without once again. However, temptation erupted and I was back to eating and drinking items made with it in a heartbeat!

Well, I told you I was an avid reader. Many books come to my attention through thoughtful friends, family and *angel-speak*. You know, when you're out shopping and you see something and that something becomes an urge, a strong urge through a voice, a thought process on your shoulder that won't let you (me) pass up a good buy. Too many times I have made purchases of last items on a store shelf, thanking my angels for their guidance. Such instances are a sure sign to me that a particular purchase is approved, encouraged. Such was the case with a book titled *Lessons from the Miracle Doctors* © 1999 by author, Jon Barron. Not only a friendly scientific read, he graciously and with brevity, thoroughly explains facts about the human body and its scores of good and bad ingested items along with the environment we presently live in and with.

Another book by friend and author Tamara Dorris called *Get Well Now!* © 2003 introduced me to a product called *stevia*. Ms. Dorris writes "The only safe sweetener is Stevia. It is a natural sweetener that comes from the shrub with the same name. Stevia is not sugar, but many times sweeter and it contains nutrients." I never heard of it before reading her book. However, I am now a faithful user. Katrina would be happy!

A newspaper article entitled "The Scoop on Sugar Substitutes" by Joy Bauer (March 1, 2009) briefly yet thoroughly compares the pink, yellow and blue packets of sweeteners with the few available stevia packets. Hands down, I'm sticking with stevia!

Author Kevin Trudeau in his *"Natural Cures They Don't Want You to Know About"* © 2004, writes a strong dialogue about the negativities of this man-made chemical, aspartame. It's awful but eye-opening! This book has opened my eyes to so many realms of man-made chemical medicines. It is frightening.

I've also learned to garnish sugar-free vanilla ice cream with various goodies such as the herb chocolate-mint which I grow, or sugar-free chocolates, grape-nuts cereal, or Rice Krispies with or without walnuts or almonds – any of a number of creative and digestible, healthy and creative ideas, are available and always within limits. Happy, creative, innovative foods and treats help to keep this diabetic person happy! It is part of taking care of me.

Without happiness, all is lost.

Having an herb garden for many years has encouraged me to be more creative with dietary needs as well as simple cures for simple symptoms such as stomach-aches, diarrhea, sore throat, headaches, ringing in the ears, etc. For instance, the sugar-free ice creams that carry chunks of nuts and/or chocolate are not encouraged due to the caloric content. Having to take extra insulin to have a bowl of ice cream just doesn't make sense to me. I might as well eat the regular stuff!

Thinking about the years and years and years and years of eating 'sugar-free,' trying to do the best I can, I have since thrown it all away. Strongly compelled and heart-broken at the same time, I threw the sugar-free (s/f) candies into the trash along with the s/f Jello, the jelly, the pancake mix, the candy bar, the gum, the sodas, and such. You get the idea. It didn't seem right to me for the longest time to be consuming this stuff. It's unnatural. I bought it and consumed it because that is what was available: dietetic for the diabetic.

Most recently I received an e-mail entitled *"Sweet Poison."* The 9-page e-mail story begins and ends in 2001. A woman's sister, diagnosed with Muscular Dystrophy (MS), became violently ill to the point of having to get around in a wheel chair. Her "medical doctors could not determine what was wrong with her. She was in so much pain, and so sick, she just knew she was dying." So, her symptoms became illogical to medical doctors.

It goes on to read how the ill sister, a diet Coke fanatic, ingested other items containing *aspartame* under the label of *sugar-free*. The sister writing this e-mail went on to write that she recalled "an article...a lawyer had sent" pertaining to aspartame being in diet sodas. The sister begged the afflicted sister to stop drinking the diet soda. As it turns out, "32 hours...after she had stopped drinking the diet soda...she could walk. She had to take a pill for the Aspartame poisoning and is well on her way to a complete recovery."

The storywriter, lecturing at the *World Environmental Conference* on the subject of aspartame goes on to write that "In the keynote address by the EPA (Environmental Protection Agency), it was announced that in the United States in 2001, there is an epidemic of multiple sclerosis and systemic lupus. It was difficult to determine exactly what toxin was causing this to be rampant."

That's it. No more for me. That e-mail was a sign! Funny 'ha-ha' or funny as in 'weird,' I'm not going to use it anymore!

Chapter 9
"You were dancing in your sleep!"

Convulsions were not strangers to me. I believe the onset of puberty with hormonal growth changes triggered such affairs. I call them "affairs" for a reason. My tongue remained scarred for many years due to my biting my tongue and trying to swallow it during such episodes. Painful, bloody messes after these episodes, it remained swollen for days after, making it difficult for me to eat, drink, swallow, and talk.

Sharing a bedroom with my younger sister, Gina, it was she who awoke my mother in the middle of those many nights due to my twitching, kicking, and snarling. One specific instance is recalled to me by my mother stating "that Gina ran down the hall one night so fast the she broke the wall light switch, screaming "Andrea's dancing, Andrea's dancing." Alarm! Through Gina, alarm was sounded throughout the house, once again.

Before the glucagon mixture via injection was introduced to combat such episodes, my mother used a mixture of orange juice and sugar, trying desperately to get this concoction down my throat. It worked on more than one occasion.

"Glucagon is a hormone that raises glucose (blood sugar) levels. It is available as a prescription medication that can be injected to resolve severe episodes of low glucose (hypoglycemia). Glucagon acts in the opposite manner of insulin, which lowers blood glucose by moving it into the body's cells. Glucagon and insulin are both naturally occurring messenger chemicals normally produced by the pancreas that are necessary to regulate glucose, the

[human] *body's* *main* *source-of-energy."*
(**http://www.diabetes.healthcenteronline.com.**)

The day after such a trauma left me feeling weak, exhausted, with my tongue torn and swollen. Well, no school for those days. As mentioned earlier, the after taste of the sugared orange juice, never mind the smell of it, was appalling to me for many years to come and it stung my tongue. The smell of orange juice made me nauseous. I just couldn't drink it. Apple juice became my choice of quick solutions to hypoglycemic reactions and remains that way to this day.

My family members were just as exhausted. Days after were spent quietly as we all tried to recover from such an emergency in those early mornings hours. Gina and my mother helped save my life.

It wasn't until many years later that an endocrinologist at the Worcester Memorial Hospital, Dr. John Stock, scheduled a brain scan for me along with a panel of fasting blood sugars. Being a new patient of his, his concern was brain damage after too many convulsions, for good reason. However, the scan was normal. Phew! But my HbA1c test was 14. Terribly bad. It should be at 6.8 or lower! HbA1c is a hemoglobin measure of chronic glucose control.

What's HbA1c and what's it mean?

"Hb = hemoglobin, the compound in the red blood cells that transports oxygen. Hemoglobin occurs in several variants; the one which composes about 90% of the total is known as hemoglobin A. A1c is a specific subtype of hemoglobin A. The 1 is actually a subscript to the A, and the c is a subscript to the 1. 'Hemoglobin' is also spelled 'haemoglobin', depending on your geographic allegiance.

Glucose binds slowly to hemoglobin A, forming the A1c

subtype. The reverse reaction, or decomposition, proceeds relatively slowly, so any buildup persists for roughly 4 weeks. Because of the reverse reaction, the actual HbA1c level is strongly weighted toward the present. Some of the HbA1c is also removed when erythrocytes (red blood cells) are recycled after their normal lifetime of about 90-120 days. These combine so that the HbA1c level represents the average bG level of approximately the past 4 weeks, strongly weighted toward the most recent 2 weeks. It is almost entirely insensitive to bG levels more than 4 weeks previous.

In non-diabetic persons, the formation, decomposition and destruction of HbA1c reach a steady state with about 3.0% to 6.5% of the hemoglobin being the A1c subtype. Most diabetic individuals have a higher average bG level than non-diabetics, resulting in a higher HbA1c level. The actual HbA1c level can be used as an indicator of the average recent bG level. This in turn indicates the possible level of glycation damage to tissues, and thus of diabetic complications, if continued for years.

Interpreting HbA1c values can be tricky for several reasons."
www.faqs.org/faqs/diabetes/faq/part2/section-9.html.

What this meant to me was that I had very important work to do to keep myself alive and feeling better. That meant paying extreme attentions to the old routine: diet, exercise, insulin, stress levels. It scared me to attention for sure!

Dr. John Stock was also the first doctor, endocrinologist, to tell me, once I asked, that my lifespan would not exceed the age of 63 – *if I was lucky.* So, here I go again, wanting to conquer the world, my world in this life, with tasks and accomplishments and trips and meetings and doings!

It wasn't long after that my older sister, Marcy, and I shared a bedroom. She witnessed one or two of these episodes herself. I don't recall. They were not pleasant for anyone involved.

"Convulsions." The word itself is awful in its self-explanatory verbiage.

Reporting to Dr. Charles Graham at the Deaconess Hospital in Brookline, Massachusetts, the outcome was for me to have a more sufficient bed-time snack. A bowl of cereal with milk, or a graham cracker - yes one graham cracker.

I continue to treat myself to peanut butter on a graham cracker, or two, which has caused me to gain weight. With this in mind, I go for a one to two mile walk. As with everything in my life, actions of any sort, especially partaking activities, depends upon how I feel and my blood sugar level. It is part of the strategic balancing act that is so very important with this disease.

At the age of eight through my mother's research, she and I began tri-monthly visits to the Deaconess Hospital where we met Dr. Graham. Although the Naval Hospital was also visited for medical supplies and groceries, the Deaconess was the top of the top for diabetes care. It still is, with the Joslin Diabetes Center right next door.

This was a time when my mother and I would be alone, just the two of us, during these car trips outside of Boston. It was delightful. We talked girl-talk. She helped me to think of other things in my life, our lives. Occasionally we treated ourselves to a Chinese lunch on the way home via Route 9. There were many such restaurants back then. Due to the high content of vegetables on such menus, mom and I felt guilt-free and glamorous together, eating globs of chow mien vegetables. I learned table manners, articulation, how to speak up [to a waiter], as well as respect of strangers. When giving respect and courtesy to others, you get it back.

Dr. Graham always got a full report of my life: school, school grades, appetite, insulin reactions, convulsions, friends, camp, and the same kids we knew, my blood sugars, my diet, my exercise routine, etc. I was honest with him and him with me. He once told me "that diabetics are smart and had good grades because they had to." I didn't understand that comment at the time and had to digest it over many months. But as usual, I concluded that he was correct. I was smart. I was an A-student. My theory is that having to strive for a better life because of diabetes was portrayed in every waking hour. I learned very young that life was work and I was going to work it!

I last visited with him in 1987 before moving to Fort Lauderdale, Broward County, Florida. Being accepted into a college in Boca Raton, Dr. Graham allowed me to interview him for an application essay I had to write. With tape recorder in hand, he treated me to lunch at a salad/sandwich shop close to the hospital. My essay was a success and I was on my way. However, I never did see Dr. Graham again. After sending him a "Thank You-for-your-time card," communication ceased. Gosh, I've missed him!

He never knew it, but I always wished he was my father.

In brief, I would like to share the following with you in memory of this wonderful man:

Charles A. Graham, M. D.

"MILLIS, MA - Dr. Charles A. Graham, 79, died Wednesday, Oct. 3, 2007, at his Millis home. He was the husband of Barbara (Blair) Graham. Born and raised in Spokane, Wash., he was the son of the late Roy A. and Mabel M. (Comstock) Graham. He received a pharmacy degree from Washington State University. Following his service during the Korean War with the Sixth Army, he attended the University of Washington, School of Medicine.

Dr. Graham served an internship and residency in internal medicine at Crawford W. Long Hospital in Atlanta, Ga., where he met his wife. Following a year's fellowship, he joined the Joslin Diabetes Center in Boston, where he spent the next 29 years directly caring for people with diabetes.

During that period, he was particularly involved with the Elliot P. Joslin Camp for boys with diabetes.

Besides his wife, he leaves five sons, William Graham and his wife, Ellen, Robert Graham and his wife, Shannon, of Millis, Richard Graham and his wife, Colleen, of Franklin, Roy Graham of Uxbridge and Timothy Graham and his wife, Laura, of Richmond Hill, Ga.; one sister, Margaret Johnson and her husband, Jack, of Spokane, Wash.; one brother, Richard Graham and his wife, Ann, of Las Vegas, Nev.; and 11 grandchildren.

Memorial donations may be made to the <u>Charles Graham Fund,</u> Joslin Diabetes Center, 1 Joslin Place, Boston, MA 02215.

Outside of my personal history, our United States was experiencing a historical upheaval, the Vietnam War. Although it is written that the U. S. involvement peaked in 1968, television news stations were constant and persistent. There was no way to get away from it, no matter where a person went. Adult conversation pertaining to this 'dilemma,' as it was phrased, was ever-present.

At the approximate age of eleven, I recall being frightened. My sixth-grade teachers requested essays on the subject. I remember writing and fulfilling these homework requests. I remember the research I used from mom's magazines and library magazines, specifically *The Times*, but I do not recall what I wrote. I do not recall what I read! I certainly did not understand that war. I did not understand the citizens' uprising at the time, the hateful displays and comments. It was not good.

This war leads to my elementary class teachings of communism, democracy, dictatorship, and the particular leaders that went with it all.

Personally, school studies went on, school dances went on, injections continued, mom's stress went on, etc.

And then there was something called *"Woodstock."* To me, Woodstock was an event of great adventure, of great fun. It was a good-to-great happening, a celebration that relieved the stress of war, a celebration of youth. I recall the full expression of the word *freedom* through the expression of America's youth through their clothes (or lack thereof), their hairstyles (or lack thereof); the use of our Constitutions' freedom of speech; the music; the drugs; the dancing through shaking their heads of hair with spastic body movements; their camping/surviving on the land; the naturalness of hundreds of thousands of humans in one spot at one time. This event impressed upon me at the time that such an undisciplined magnitude of adults could behave so erratically and irresponsibly! It seemed like fun!

Sure, I had a fleeting thought about being there. Just a thought. But reality shook my soul. For one, I knew I was too young. Second, where would I put my insulin? Third, I was a strict Catholic-school girl under strict management of body, soul and mind. However, imagine…

Chapter 10
Oh no, not her!

One fall day, October 16th to be exact, I tumbled into the house after school. Mom's car was there, unusual for any day. It turns out that my kid sister, Judy, was sitting on my mother's lap, crying. Diagnosed with diabetes on this day in 1969, her fifth birthday, mom looked to me for support. My being twelve years old at the time, I tried my best to console this youngest of siblings, sharing with her the many plans of how I would help take care of her. But I wouldn't give her a shot. At least not in the beginning. Mom had to do that. "And maybe she could go to camp with me and learn how to give her own shot, just like I did," I cried. I was serious. I wanted her to share the camp life happiness with me. I wanted her to feel the happiness, the joy I felt there!

Well, that plan came to fruition, briefly. Timid, shy, Judy did not like camp life. A petite, fair skinned tow-head of a child with transparent blue eyes, she allowed herself to spend only one summer at CBC. I was disappointed. However, she did learn how to give herself her shots. That took a load off of my mind because I really did not want to have to do that!

In the meantime, I continued summer sessions at CBC. I would have stayed longer if they let me. I went so far as to become a Councilor-In-Training (CIT). That last summer, Lisa K., Cathy C., Diane C., Buffy, Laurie W., Judy V. some others I can't remember, and I, shared our experiences and knowledge as older campers by becoming CITs. It was basically a voluntary babysitting position, but the respect and reward were worth the efforts. At age 13, I greatly looked forward to helping the little ones, the young campers, learn how to take care of themselves. I was to be a good example! I was proud of this opportunity and myself! After all, my experience having to take care of younger siblings at home as well as myself gave me background experience and knowledge of what, when, why, where, how, and how much to do anything!

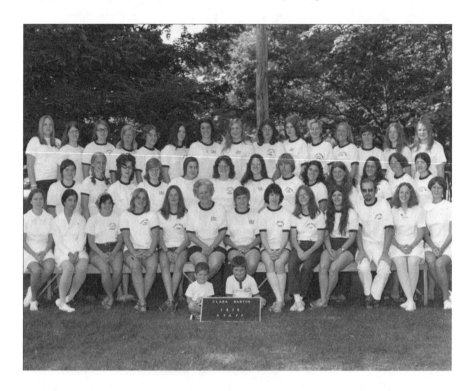

Adult supervision was relaxed with CITs. More than a few CITs took advantage of this attitude and walked the three miles to and from a nearby General Store. Among its many items, the passionate craving for regular candy was appeased. I was witness to occasions of a few of my buddies walking up there and indulging themselves with sugar loaded treats. Well, Judy V. got so sick that she had to be taken to a hospital. Of course, the rest of us worried in silence. Not only was this secret out about the excursion to the 'candy store,' but we had to betray our friend in order to save her life. Chastised by our counselors, we were branded as breaking an unwritten law. Shame amassed each of us, innocent or guilty.

Back a few days later, Judy V. proclaimed that her blood sugar reached 1600! Definite ketoacidosis. Her blood was turning into acid. That's what happens. An explanation follows:

> *"Diabetic ketoacidosis (DKA) is a dangerous condition that occurs when a severe lack of insulin causes the body to break down fats instead of glucose (blood sugar) for energy. This process can cause waste products called ketones to build up in the blood. If untreated, DKA can lead to diabetic coma or death. However, with proper medical treatment, patients can recover from DKA and prevent it from recurring. Ketoacidosis may develop because of an infection or illness. This condition may also develop when people fail to properly control their diabetes, as a result of pregnancy complications or from an eating disorder. DKA is more common with type 1 diabetes, although it can affect those with type 2 diabetes. The American Diabetes Association estimates that DKA is responsible for 10 percent of all diabetes–related deaths for diabetic individuals under the age of 45.*

> *"DKA develops because of three factors: Severe lack of insulin; Very high levels of glucose; and Very high levels of ketones.*

> *"The typical treatment options for DKA are intravenous (I.V.) treatments and replacing lost insulin. Patients can reduce their risk of DKA by: Adhering to their diet plan; Taking insulin as prescribed; and Monitoring glucose and performing ketone tests; Making a sick-day plan; Taking precautions against infections and injuries; and Ensuring caregivers' education."*
> **(http://diabetic.healthcentersonline.com.)**

My personal experience with acquiring regular candies while at CBC did not involve the General Store. I thought I was going to be smarter! Before Judy V.'s excursion and episode, I wrote a friend of mine back home for her to please send me some candy. Well, when the package came, brimming with such items as raisinettes, jujubees, and bubble gum, it was opened before I got it. To my horror, a camp counselor confiscated the stuff and called my mother. I was in so-oo-o much trouble. Yelled at, grounded, reduced to a thumb tack via telephone, I did not want to go home after session ended! I tested the authorities at hand, as teenagers will do, got caught, thank goodness, and accepted my punishment. From that day forward, the CIT lounge was closed down. A padlock placed on the door dramatized our mischievous behavior. That was the example we left for the younger campers: outlandish behavior is not only intolerable but unacceptable as well.

Not being able to take back what was done, the incident was not forgotten, but faded away. We averted our energies toward whatever it was we were supposed to be doing anyway such as laundry, cleaning our tents, and/or straightening the rocks on the path leading to wherever. As CIT's, we were given privileges to the laundry facility in the barn, as long as a counselor wasn't using them. One washer and one dryer were available, so we had to scurry when they were available and make sure we had time to stay with our clothes. If we wanted the hand laundry service to take care of our stuff as when we were little, a price had to be paid. On a strict budget as it was, my mother did not deem it necessary to add such a quota to my allowance.

You see, as little children campers, it was a requirement that all our belongings, including all clothes articles, be labeled before we left home. I don't recall if the ever-popular *Sharpie* markers were available back then, but I do recall using a black marker to write my initials on everything I was taking. Once settled at camp, each camper was provided a laundry bag for soiled clothing, of course. Once that was filled, it was sent out for laundering with the multitude of all the other campers' bags. That's why it was so-oo-o important to have name labels on *everything,* especially your clothes! Too many times I witnessed children missing clothes items or their items being mixed up with another child's. I never had that problem.

A year later, my sister Gina was diagnosed with diabetes. The fourth sibling and third sister, the second to the youngest, she was twelve years old at the time. Already dealing with scoliosis, embarrassment at having to wear a specially designed back brace for her little body was an additional specialty. Gina did not look at these issues as burdens. She shrugged her shoulders and said "That's the way it is." The brace accompanied her during her two summers at CBC where she met another girl, a little older, who had gone through a specific and delicate spinal-pin surgery successfully. No matter how cumbersome and awkward, Gina was told that the specific corrective surgery offered to her and available at the time carried a 30% - 70% ratio of full recuperation. With this fact in mind, Gina did not succumb to surgery and wore that brace until she was twenty years old. It was used to help straighten her spine, keeping certain back muscles in place where they belong. This also brought her chronic, irritating pain.

Extremely active, thin in stature, square- shouldered and quick, she was our family's childhood "tom boy." Most importantly, she was our brothers' pal. Those two high-spirited youngsters were always in some secretive plan together: either roaming a field, building a clubhouse, figuring out a gadget or a tool.

Gina did go on to college and graduated as a Medical Technician and Transcriptionist. Chucky also went on to college with physics as his main interest. However, Gina's career was cut short due to retinopathy.

> **"Diabetic retinopathy** *is retinopathy (damage to the retina) caused by complications of diabetes mellitus, which can eventually lead to blindness. It is an ocular manifestation of systemic disease which affects up to 80% of all patients who have had diabetes for 10 years or more. Despite these intimidating statistics, research indicates that at least 90% of these new cases could be reduced if there was proper and*

vigilant treatment and monitoring of the eyes."

With her limited eyesight, she accepted a live-in, caretaking position for an elderly woman. After a few months of Gina's getting into this new job routine, the home owners decided to re-roof the house. As the old woman napped, Gina stepped out into the backyard to clean the pool after the workers' had left. While getting some fresh air and sun, she stepped on a rusty nail left haphazardly by the unkempt workers. This accident brought on a foot infection which began agonizing months of physical pain and mental anxiety.

Facing amputation, she checked herself out of the Deaconess Hospital in Brookline, Massachusetts, to care for herself and this wound in her "home element."

Also dealing with gastrointestinal neuropathy, this wiry, energetic and beautiful young woman became paralyzed from the waist down. She was in constant pain and taking so many prescription medications that I couldn't count them. The medication display on her bedroom bureau constantly reminded me of the collection of medication I saw while employed as a Home Health Care Worker with Catholic Charities and being a Visiting Nurses Aide many years before.

But Gina wasn't old!

At the age of 23, she was partially blind and became confined to her bed.

"Gastrointestinal symptoms are relatively common among patients with diabetes and often reflect diabetic gastrointestinal autonomic neuropathy. The prevalence of symptoms caused by gastrointestinal dysfunction may reach 76% in a non-selected population of diabetic outpatients. Esophageal dysfunction results at least in part from vagal neuropathy; symptoms include heartburn and dysphagia for solids.

...Diarrhea and other lower gastrointestinal tract symptoms may also occur. Diabetic diarrhea manifests as a profuse,

watery, typically nocturnal diarrhea, which can last for hours or days and frequently alternates with constipation. Abdominal discomfort is commonly associated. The pathogenesis of diabetic diarrhea includes reduced gastrointestinal motility, reduced receptor mediated fluid absorption, bacterial overgrowth, pancreatic insufficiency, coexistent celiac disease, and abnormalities in bile salt metabolism. Fecal incontinence due to anal sphincter incompetence or reduced rectal sensation is another manifestation of diabetic gastrointestinal neuropathy. The most common problem associated with diabetic gastrointestinal dysfunction is constipation, affecting nearly 60% of diabetic patients. Severe constipation may be complicated by perforation and fecal impaction."
(www.medscape.com.)

With not wanting to leave this elderly woman out of assistance, my mother and I split Gina's shifts and duties in between my college course schedule and mom's full-time job.

Feisty, determined, and strong-willed, Gina was bound and determined to get better. She tried to be like other 23 year olds – she tried to be "normal." To dream, to continue college, have a boyfriend, get married, and be happy.

Eugenia Marie died at the age of 26. The coroner's report reads "heart attack." I think it was a broken heart. She fought all her short life for her life and she didn't win the war. The year was 1986.

If it wasn't for my sister, Gina, having babysat for my daughter during my five years of night classes at Worcester State College, it would have been much more difficult as a single mother. Gina and Heather loved each other deeply and genuinely as a niece/aunt relationship should be. Heather misses her as well as all of those who knew this charming and comedic young woman. Heather and Gina were good for each other. Gina was a good sister. Gina was a good person. She was there for me. Her lively soul couldn't take any more pain. I understand, truly. Although it took me a few years, I finally let her spirit go into the hands of God. She is no longer in pain. Such is my eulogy to Gina. She will continue to be missed. The photograph of Gina depicts her presenting me a birthday cake on my 30th birthday earlier that year. Thank you, Gina.

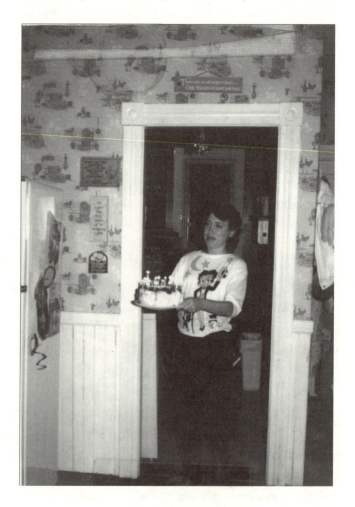

Not only a single parent of five, mom not only had to cope with three diabetics, but now the heart-wrenching death of a child.

Judy? She went on to her second year of college when diabetes complications set in. Having developed retinopathy, laser treatments were to no avail when she lost her eyesight completely at age 28. This further lead to her having kidney failure resulting in a kidney transplant in 1994. Judy did marry, in 1996.

She and Karl first met because of me. One summer, I was dating a young man and she wanted to hang around with me that day and go with me to meet him. My date, awestruck by our resemblance, repeatedly cajoled his roommate to wake up, come downstairs, and meet us. It was Karl.

Judy and Karl, also diabetic, met again many years later in a dialysis support group at UMass. They couldn't see each other because of their blindness, of course, but they liked each other, had too many commonalities, and eventually wed. Before their wedding, however, I happened to visit with them. Intervening, I helped Judy and Karl recollect that, in fact, they did meet, they did actually "see" each other at one time! "Oh my gosh, Judy," Karl exclaimed. "You're that gorgeous blonde that was sitting under the window at my old roommate's house. How do you like that? Your hair was so long, and beautiful and shiny! Ahh, I remember! No kidding! I'm marrying the most beautiful girl in the world!" And such was their love.

Through Karl's diabetes complications, he passed away in 2005 at the age of 44. Judy remains living in the home that she and Karl shared. Judy and I continue to reminisce about camp, some of the same acquaintances - and Karl. They are fond ones, tremendously fond.

Due to her blindness, I became involved with the *Hadley School for the Blind* in Chicago, Illinois. My purpose was to learn Braille in order to communicate with Judy but also as a foreboding for myself. With two sisters having gone blind due to diabetes, it seems inevitable that this would happen to me. Therefore, with a little planning and lots of practice, I became acquainted with the Braille language.

Having visited camp on numerous occasions, without a trace of another human being, I was delighted to walk the premises, reminiscing. I never stayed very long, perhaps 30 minutes. I did not want to be arrested for trespassing! Often, visits were covered in snow and the glee I felt just to be there was overwhelming, amassed in a gorgeous coverlet of white. Thoughts of the place always bring me peace of mind, a sense of hope that encourages happiness.

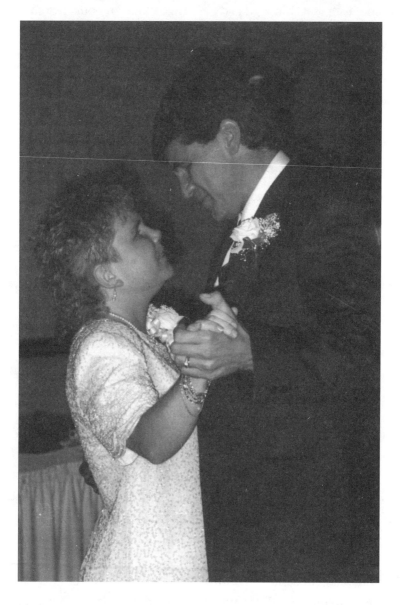

I continue to donate monetarily to their cause. In turn, I receive *The Barton Spirit* aka: *The Barton Center* newsletter every quarter. The background pictures along with its stories are most enjoyable and reminiscent to me and will continue to be. I miss that place; I miss my childhood there, I miss my sisters and my brother. Therefore, the **10% profit-sharing** of this book is important to me and completely justified. CBC is in my soul.

Chapter 11
Heard that, been there, done it.

Throughout the early '70's, great news befell the world that a cure for diabetes was closely on the horizon. I paid that announcement no heed. I couldn't remember how many times I had heard that same briefing. I could never count how many times newspaper articles boasted about a cure as those previously shown on behind page 28. I no longer collect those headlines. My mother, another family member, or a friend will always ask if I had read a certain article or seen a certain TV commercial pertaining to diabetes therapy. If not, I humor them into explaining it to me. It gives people pleasure to know that they have hope for me, for the general public concerning this epidemic.

Nowadays there are pamphlets located at pharmaceutical sections pertaining to diabetes and diabetes only. They are insights into managing this disease. There are so many of them that I find them rather overwhelming. Just the thought of so many separate articles, separate pamphlets, frightens me with the ever-present reality of this expensive pandemic. I find that the marketing and advertising of the disease and its accoutrements quite shameful. Some pamphlets, quick-reads, have even been located at grocery stores. They write about the gamut of involvements concerning this disease from warning signs, the treatments, the expectations, the complications on a one-page, two-sided sheet of brochure paper to the hopeful possibilities and thoughts of a cure. Some are thicker. One particular information booklet titled *"A Guide to Living Well with Diabetes: Inner Strength* (2006) excitedly proclaimed a "breakthrough." It introduces the drug "Symlin." Writer Oona Short gives us a two-paragraph article proclaiming the possibility of eradicating this disease through a vaccine. And of course there are cookbooks available alongside the ever popular media magazines located at the checkout. As I wait in line at a check-out counter, as I'm sure you have done, a whole magazine can be read just by their cover titles. There is always a special cookbook for diabetics. I don't like it, the propagandizing, profiteering of a serious, and life threatening matter.

Well, glory be! Eradication. Isn't that what I want to hear?! Isn't that what I want, what I would like to see? However, and once again, I've been hearing and reading such upcoming, futuristic possibilities all my life. And I will continue to see them, view them, notice them, but I won't read them. The articles and their catchy titles are fascinating if only because so many people are involved with the same concentrated goal – getting rid of *it*, abdicating *it* from society. This way, hope is kept alive.

How physically simple this disease has been made to appear. Yet the glossy advertising is costly along with all aspects of this disease. I feel that diabetes, along with so many terminal diseases, has come to financially support this country. I'll discuss that further along.

And so it was that same year, 1970, that I was told by an insurance agent whom was meeting with my mother at our house that I would be lucky to see the age of 31. Not a happy thing to digest at the age of 12. This news took me many frightening years to recover. I was in a hurry to grow, to learn, to accomplish; in a hurry to try things, good or bad; in a hurry to go places; in a hurry to meet as many people as I could; in a hurry to read as many books as I could; in a hurry to be remembered; a hurry to make an impression. I wanted so much to be special. However, I carried on. Continued to do what all 12-year olds do. Bike-ride, babysit for siblings and others, read, daily chores, summer camp. And I loved to write letters. A collection of special pen-pals from CBC kept me busy. I concentrated on my studies, as I was a good student. And I took care of my diabetes as I was taught. Dr. Graham not only told me "that diabetics are smarter than other kids." But he went on to say that "you're the only one that will ever know your disease. Don't let anyone kid you." He was right, in more ways than one!

My Diabetic Soul

While spending summers at CBC, I had met one other family with three children being diabetic. They were the Mars family. Surprising to me, our families didn't communicate. We were not stirred by similarities or encouraged to contact each other. I never understood the ineptitude of attitudes from either side. I lost contact when I outgrew CBC.

Adolescence. This period was such a busy part of my life's story. The worst and the best if only because of the lessons learned. Among facts of peer pressure and making decisions for my personal welfare, decisions, difficult decisions had to be made. Adolescence, my adolescence, was a sojourn into the world.

I was a run-away at the age of 17½. After a *terrible* argument with my mother one early morning in September, 1974, before leaving for school, I stormed out of the house. I got in my '62 Ford Fairlane and went to the room where my older sister rented and lived. Already a high school graduate, she was on her way to establishing her life, independently.

When I walked into her unlocked studio apartment, she immediately began yelling – no, screaming – at me for showing up there. Just behind me was our mother with insulin and syringes in hand, saying something to the effect that "if this is how you want to live, take your stuff and go." Well I did. Evidently, I got through it. I phrase this period of my life 'as the first adventure into realistic and frightening independence '

Well, knowing I was not wanted at Marcy's, I got back in my car and went to school. I was always a good student, maintained excellent grades and wanted to be there. The '62 Ford was acquired during that last summer from my mother's boss for $1.00. He wanted it off his property. And since I had gloriously passed the driving test, I was good to go.

Well, my stubbornness and I slept in that car until pay day when I bought a newspaper to look for a place to live. That experience lasted all of a chilly 3 days. With the insulin and syringes I had, I was able to inject what I was used to injecting each day while sitting in my car. I ate at the grocery store where I worked, indulging myself with food from behind the deli-counter.

I found a room for rent. $50.00 a week got me a bedroom in a private home off Pleasant Street with a communal bathroom and refrigerator in an acceptably nice neighborhood. With two other roommates whom I never saw, my third of the refrigerator hid my insulin and syringes along with some scant groceries (eggs, milk, bread, butter and celery, of course). Although those groceries cost me $10.00 at the time, that ten dollars was a big expense for me.

This arrangement also gave me another job which cut my rent in half. Due to the 92-year old home owner living there, he needed to be watched, cared for, and basically kept company during evening hours. I took the position which was delightful if only because I could sit with him, study, read aloud to his enjoyment, and keep him company. He enjoyed it as well. He always smiled at me and listened intently to my readings until he fell asleep. He also told me to indulge myself in the antique books that he kept close at hand. I still have those books, written by *Robert Lewis Stevenson* in 1902.

After two weeks of living there, a high school friend one year ahead of me invited me to live with her and her family. Heck, they lived up the street from my mother who decided not to have anything to do with me. Nothing! She called the cops on me one time when I went to visit my siblings and I almost got arrested for trespassing! Because of that instance, I didn't see my siblings for a *very* long time. I really can't recall how long that was. I estimate between two and three years. Seriously. It was awful.

Even though we went to the same school, I never saw them, even when I looked for them. I was bad for running away. They were frightened. This was a very sad situation.

In the meantime, I graciously and without hesitation joined a Choir Group with this live-in family. The mother played along with my friend, her oldest child. There was a third guitar player and a tambourine handler. I was one of many singers. Being able to reach high soprano notes, I was a welcome part of the group. Meeting at St. Mark's Cathedral every Saturday night kept me busy and out of trouble. It was a pleasurable experience wherein I could use the beautiful voice God gave me to sing in one of His houses.

Yes, I finished putting myself through St. Mary's Parochial High School. Working part time after school in a grocery store as a deli clerk, then as a cashier, I slimly supported myself. Tuition at the time was $250.00 a month. I paid it. Come to find out many years later, my mother was paying my tuition as well. The school authorities never said a thing. I still can't believe it. And there I was thinking that mom would have extra money for the three younger kids at home. That job lasted for 2 ½ years until I graduated.

Purposely close to my sister's place, I rented another studio apartment down the street for $23.00 a week. It was the autumn of 1974. The kitchen, bath, pay telephone, laundry facility, and mail box were communal. Parking was 'grab it if you see it.' Having a 1962 Buick LeSabre that I bought for $200.00; it was difficult finding a parking spot because of the size of that car. During snow storms it was worse, a lot worse! There were too many times when I had no other choice than to park in the nearby, empty church lot. The car was never towed; however, more than a few times it was buried under many of feet of snow while the rest of the lot was clear. I still think that that act of unkind spite will be claimed to the fate of the person(s) who did that to me. What goes around comes around! Because it took me hours and hours to dig out of that snow mound, I was late for work, late for school, etc. I could never be so spitefully unkind to anyone like that. Lesson learned, a lesson in compassion.

Sooner or later, in between school, school studies, work, and 'band practice,' I was introduced to parties wherein alcohol and marijuana were rampant. After all, I now had my own place. There was always someone around that wanted to hang out and old enough to buy the beer or whatever. I welcomed the company. But the easily-gotten- and consumed-beer made me hungry. Since I couldn't afford "hungry,' such instances didn't happen too often. It wasn't until many years later that I read how alcoholic beverages quickly raise, and then as quickly lower a diabetic's blood sugar level. Thank goodness for my collection of sugar packets from co-worker's ordering coffees. Once too often a few of those were eaten in the wee morning hours due to an insulin reaction. That's all I had.

Breakfasts, yes, but rarely. Cream cheese and bagels were gotten at work the next morning at 6:00am. I swear that's the only reason I went to work. The other kids, my co-workers, just *knew* I'd be hungry! I always was.

And to hell with the urine testing. I knew it wouldn't be good. I went many – no, many more – years denying that that procedure was a controlling factor. I didn't want to be controlled. Although I continued my daily regime of two insulin shots per day, I knew to lower the dosages due to how I "felt." I was invincible, an attitudinal mindset for all teenagers.

If I was tired, shaky, sweaty and weak, especially all at once, I diagnosed myself as hypoglycemic and lowered the insulin amount. If I was thirsty, dry-skinned, bad breath, tired and grumpy all at the same time, that meant I needed more insulin.

Geez, what a game I played with my life!

Taking on extra hours at the grocery store further helped me to support myself. With my United States Naval Identification card, I was able to get my prescriptions when needed – insulin and syringes, always insulin and syringes. Such a trip necessitated a day off from school. Gasoline for the car meant I had to sacrifice *something* when I didn't have anything, really. At the time, gas was 0.23 – yes, 23 cents – a gallon, which further dates me. However, I dug it up from somewhere because I needed to take that one hour trip to get that darn insulin!

When asked for a parent's note at school, I continued to ignore the request until Mother Superior knew not to bother asking. She had already telephoned my mother and they must have had one heck of a conversation! What developed was an implied agreement of sorts, like a fog around me, that lead to my not being bothered. Emancipation at that time was unheard of, never mind attending an elite private/parochial school. Because I was accused of breaking one of God's commandments, "Honor Thy Father and Thy Mother," I was further ostracized. High school friendships were rare and fleeting. Although I was the first kid to have a car during my junior and senior years, it was purposely used for school, work and home. I couldn't afford to joy-drive kids here and there. They stopped asking after a while.

Food was scarce. There were more than a couple of times that all I could afford was cat food. I ate it if only to satiate myself. Another staple was chicken livers. It was better tasting than cat food, but more expensive. Working at the grocery store helped to sustain me further if not cause me to gain an exorbitant amount of weight after a time. Totally out of sight of any diet control, cream cheese with bagels from the delicatessen I served was gratefully consumed – if and when I could get them. And that was only if a co-worker was treating. I know they felt sorry for me. Many of the kids were struggling college students with limited incomes. I'm forever thankful for whatever crumbs came my way.

But, I'll be damned if I couldn't afford myself. My pride was at stake, never mind my well-being, my organs. I never asked anyone for help. I never even thought of going "home." I was going to do this all by myself with stubbornness to boot! I would take care of me. Anyway, no one knew that I was "a diabetic." Most people didn't know what that was if only "she can't eat sugar." That is where the understanding stopped – such an understatement.

Ignorance was rampant and I, in my newfound freedom, took it for granted.

Dating was fun except for the part where food was concerned. And there was always the issue of my needing to give myself a shot or the desperation of needing sugar.

The boys I went out with always wanted to go to McDonald's or get an ice cream after 9:00pm, after the movie or the ice skating rink closed. That's where one of my diabetes management boundaries broke. You see, they didn't know I was (am) an insulin dependent diabetic. They didn't have to know. All they wanted to do was have fun, maybe impress a pretty girl – me!

I knew better than to eat such high calorie foods that late at night, but I did it anyway. I wanted to fit in. If my dates knew I was diabetic, they didn't understand the personal consequences I would have to deal with in the first place. In the second place, I was sure they would not go out with me again. So I never told them. It just wasn't discussed. In fact, many boys never even knew I had to take insulin shots or carried my insulin and syringes with me in my pocket book (aka: purse, handbag, sack) 24/7.

After dating a young man for a few weeks, he asked me to go to a concert on Cape Cod. Of course I said yes! Cape Cod is one of the best places in Massachusetts to be at any time and for anything!

Arrangements were made and I was ready. To my surprise, he invited two of his buddies. All right, I could deal with that. There was room in the back seat. We were all just happy to be going to "the Cape."

On the way there, one of the guys lit up a joint (aka: marijuana cigarette). He passed it to me and I said no; the same for my date. Well, not five minutes later police sirens and lights are flashing right behind us. Good God. My date was freaking out, of course, not knowing what he did wrong. The Massachusetts State Trooper that pulled us over firmly told all of us to exit the vehicle. We did. The guys were to stand facing the car with their hands on the hood. I was to stand with my back against the passenger door of the car. Nobody moved.

After the officers' car search revealed a pouch of marijuana, the officer walked over to the side of the wooded area at the soft shoulder of the highway and dumped it out. He just let it float in the breeze, never to be had again.

The guys that had brought the dope were yelling and complaining – to the State Cop (aka: "Statey") mind you. That was disrespectful in itself! My date and I stayed quiet and watched. This officer also confiscated a bottle of booze, brandy I believe, and dumped that out on the road shoulder as well.

Then he came over to me, telling me to hand him my pocket book. I did. He found the baggie of syringes with a vial of insulin and alcohol swabs. When pulling it out and displaying it, the boys all gasped, denying they knew I had this in my possession, thinking I was a drug addict. Well, they didn't know too much of anything, really. They didn't have to. I explained to the cop that I was diabetic and that was why the syringes were there. After he examined the vial of insulin, he took the loot and walked back to his cruiser.

The ten minutes that the officer was gone, I quickly explained to the boys about being diabetic and what was in that Baggie was my medicine, my insulin. They were shocked. I was embarrassed. My date quickly changed his attitude from grief to sympathy.

The reason we were pulled over was because of the joint. Gosh, that cop had good eyes! In the end, my date received a citation and we were back on the road to the concert. The guys in the back seat just hemmed and hawed and complained the whole rest of the way as if they weren't to blame for any of this trouble. What jerks!

Now we're two hours late to this concert. Traffic was also a nuisance along with trying to find a place to park. Once having done so, the parking spot was quite a walking distance from the concert area entrance. For some reason or another, we were all denied entrance. What a bother! My date and I stayed together for the rest of that afternoon and evening while his buddies took off. We never met up with them again that day or night. My date and I never dated again, however we did see each other in passing, only to say hello to each other. The subject of our "Statey Encounter" never came up again. Neither did the topic of my diabetes.

That is one of those life instances I will *never* forget!

In short, diabetes was an embarrassment to me.

Through that ordeal, my already-low-self-confidence was lower. But that resolve was not the only reason. Diabetes was one thing I never mentioned, publicly or privately. It wasn't until intimacy entered a relationship that I allowed myself to be totally honest. I always felt *it* was too difficult to discuss to or with the other party, be it a date or a friend. It was too difficult for them to truly understand or appreciate the intricacies of this disease. When becoming close to someone, friend or relative, the innumerable questions were aggravating and relentless to me. Sure, I understood that he or she was interested. But read a book already! However, there were no books available on the subject matter. It wasn't a popular "thing." It wasn't a trend. It was and is a life-threatening disease.

"How come you can eat/drink that…(whatever) being diabetic and all?" someone would ask.

"Well," I would begin my exercised explanation, "because I substituted this for that. Also, I increased my insulin amount in order to digest this stuff."

"How do you know how much insulin to take?" someone would ask.

"I just do" would be my reply.

And that was true. I just knew, automatically, without hesitation, how many units to draw into the syringe. If that wasn't enough after ingesting something, my body signs – thirst, dry mouth, fatigue – would encourage a shot. If I took too much, once again my body signs – sweating, shaking, and not thinking clearly – would tell me I needed sugar or something with a base of quick acting calories. Apple juice has always been a personal favorite; or a half a can of regular soda would level me off for a while. Sure, sometimes I over did it, other times it's not enough, resulting in a meal or a snack with crackers, a carbohydrate base.

In the long run, I never voluntarily introduced my diabetes to anyone. I always thought to take care of it myself. *It* was my problem. I chose the secret to remain a secret. Only when I would need an emergent refresh, be it insulin or food, would I *have to* interrupt whatever it was that was going on.

Through college applications and after high school graduation, I attended part-time, evening classes at Quinsigamond Community College in Westboylston, Massachusetts. With a few 'major' changes, I settled on studies toward a Registered Nurses' degree and worked full time during the day. The factory job I was involved with allowed me to afford a one-bedroom apartment with a full kitchen and my own bathroom. Hurrah!

My Diabetic Soul

One weekend night, and with the coaching of a friend, I met and dated a man that I ended up marrying. A dream come true! And I don't just mean him – I mean the whole idea of marriage! Someone was actually interested in me, wanted to marry me! We were in love/lust. As mushy as it sounds, it was time to settle down.

As my fiancée was a non-practicing Protestant and I a semi-devote-Catholic, we were invited to attend a pre-marital interview with one of the attending priests. These days, no matter your religion or non-religion, a mandatory six-week course is available and scheduled for the proponents on the subject of marriage, discouraging divorce, before a couple is able to wed in a Catholic Church. I was adamant about a gloriously huge ceremony in – where else? – Our Lady of Częstochowa, of course. That meant that we *had* to attend this meeting. To my recollections, my fiancée and I spent approximately and hour and a half with this certain priest.

We were each asked a lot of questions, especially personal questions pertaining to our sex life. We didn't lie. But the priest didn't like our answers either. We were deemed sinners, once again, having partaken in pre-marital sex. The subject of birth control was argued, my fiancée trying to defend my health issues as the priest insisted we reproduce. What a conundrum!

With that being accomplished into a win-win situation, we were married in April of 1978 by that same interviewing priest. My life seemed to be blessed. The ever pressing thought that I just may make it to my 31st birthday was a deciding factor toward this marriage. I prayed that I would. I prayed a lot! I was happy and looked forward to being happy with my future husband. At the age of 21, I gravely knew the possible concept of leaving a husband a widower. Heck, I was a realist before knowing the definition.

However, I know he appreciated knowing that there were (are) depths to this disease and how progressively worse it can get over time. He watched my sisters get ill due to diabetes. It was me that did not realize the impact that diabetes would have on our lives together. For better or worse!

Chapter 12
The Bride has come and gone. Move on.

Children?

"Sure, I love kids. I wouldn't mind having three. But I don't think I could or should."

Too many times this subject came up. Not so much between my husband and me but with his parents, his relatives, aunts, uncles, sister, brothers, friends. Yikes! It became apparent to me, through hindsight, that our personal lives, especially mine, were not respected. Sure, it's one thing to be a concerned parent, but enough is enough after a while!

They knew I was diabetic, but they didn't understand or appreciate the depths of this disease. Even when I had gone through some real rough and unhealthy episodes, the subject of having children surfaced. Their ignorance annoyed me. It was useless to talk to them, to try and explain my heartfelt concerns with this disease. Not only was I protecting my life, but that of their sons.'

What was so wrong with my answer? Why did they pursue making me uncomfortable?

Even after my fourth pregnancy and miscarriage, my husband and I resigned to knowing that we would not have children. My body with diabetes was too fragile. My *life* would definitely be at stake. My college classes were suffering and finally postponed. I was losing interest in a once longed-for nursing career.

Both from large families, I felt the subtle anger and disappointment from my in-laws. I felt I was a failure. They made me feel like I was a failure.

I never shared the miscarriages with my immediate family. They would not approve of my childbearing in the first place. They knew the consequences, especially my mother, a Licensed Practical Nurse (LPN) at the time. My family also thought they knew that grievous consequences would strike me. I did as well. The consequences were high, too high, and too scary.

"You'll die." "You'll have to have a kidney transplant." "You'll end up in a coma!"

Oh my gosh, I grew up hearing those comments many times along with "What are you thinking?"

Well, it happened again - my fifth pregnancy.

The inclusion of my personal journal follows within a few pages. These italicized twenty-six pages were written and saved purposely for the right time to share with you, dear reader. It is the actual journal I wrote during this pregnancy. Pauses occur due to explanations that I need to share with you. It is important to me that I share this journal with you, especially the other diabetic women who have gone through diabetic pregnancies or those that plan to. It is re-written, unedited from my original manuscript. I have never shared this succinctly with anyone, although few people know of its existence. I am delighted to share it with you, dear reader, in length.

First Journal Entry:

December 30, 1980

Dr. Karen Green's secretary, Doreen, telephoned to tell me that the blood and urine tests are positive. I am pregnant.

"Congratulations!" she declared

The only thing being is that I am not very cheery about these test results. Don't know if I want to go through this – again.

My first pregnancy resulted in a miscarriage after 2½ months. The cause was 'uncontrollable blood sugars.' With the second, I was happily along when in the fourth month life stopped. Given the term 'intra-urinal fetal demise,' it meant fetal self-destruction – suicide. A ghastly thought.

Try to imagine how the planning and wondering and expectations had suddenly and quite abruptly ceased. Being that far along, I had purchased a few articles of clothing and even started putting aside jars of baby food and diapers. I ended up giving it all away.

The third pregnancy, at six weeks, ended as an abortion through a choice of my husband's and mine. No discouragement from the medical community. At this stage in my life as a diabetic, a full-term pregnancy seemed impossible.

Yes, birth control methods were in constant use. Diaphragms, jellies that caused infections, prophylactics, but not "the pill." The pill would have adverse effects on my diabetic body system. Abstinence with newlyweds was unheard of between us. It would not happen.

Once again, abortion was greatly encouraged before the 'automatic' termination of a fourth pregnancy at 2½ months – again. The term "fetal destruction" was brought into clear focus with this decision.

Having already used an IUD (Intra Uterine Device), it had to be surgical removed due to complications. When trying another of different design and manufacture, I nonetheless became pregnant and lost. Surprise, surprise! Virility was in charge between these ages of 21 - 23!

Furthermore, the awkwardness and embarrassment of spermicidal jellies and creams was ignored and their use was profound, usually resulting in an intra-urinal or painful bladder infection.

Along with the D&Cs (dilation & curettage) that followed and were performed with these miscarriages, I believed wholeheartedly in my mind that I would *never* get pregnant again! There was too much intra-uretal scar tissue, there had to be!

However, this spirit wanted to be born! A fifth and successful pregnancy resulted in our Heather Dawn. Born five weeks early through a Caesarean section, she has been considered a miracle, my miracle. But this did not happen without great painstaking and special care with lots of self-devoted time. I became adamantly selfish. I had to be in order to maintain my life's health and that of this fetus.

At this time, I don't mind sharing that Heather's earthly spirit has continued with strength, persistence, perseverance and great determination.

Before she was born I did in fact continue college courses at *Quinsig* (Quinsigamond Community College). I was able to accomplish two courses while pregnant. Unemployed, I began selling Avon Products, walking my neighborhood streets every few days to pass out catalogues, pick up orders, meet neighbors, and get exercise that is so important. It was actually fun! Avon allowed me to be out and about, accomplishing personal tasks, resting and talking and selling and encouraging others which positively contributed to my overall health and positive attitude. Multi-tasking with a sense of accomplishment was, and remains to be, a large aspect of my personality.

My profits went toward college tuition and supplies, meaning the expensive textbooks. Selling Avon products padded my $20.00 week allowance that I received from my husband. Yes, I scrimped and did it well!

My sister-in-law at the time gave me most, if not all, of her maternity clothes. The bathing suit was the best thing. It got a lot of use. That saved me money, as well, big money. Glad to have taken a sewing class many years prior, I was able to sew a few items for myself, trying to be stylish and pregnant.

My long-term, juvenile diabetes and bi-annual follow-ups with the Joslin Diabetes Foundation in Boston proved that my health was attended to properly if only because of having better medical insurance through my husband's employer. At one point I had been contacted about a new program for the 'pregnant diabetic.' This would include family planning for the diabetic woman planning to bear children.

The program consisted of learning how to use an insulin pump machine that is strapped to one hip or the other (see photograph next page). Before hand, I had never heard of such a device. My curiosity was peaked. Thoughts of being a guinea pig, a human experiment for the welfare of all diabetics entered my mind. I had to find out more. I had to learn what science was offering me and perhaps the rest of the world.

With the use of a transparent tube and a micro-fine needle at one end, the needle is inserted under the skin and thus releases small doses of insulin throughout a 24-hour period. Having called a few months earlier due to curiosity, it was certainly a good thing I put my name of the waiting list!

Due to the insistent and persistent care of certain special and attentive doctors closer to home such as Dr. Karen G., OB/GYN Specialist at what is now known as the Worcester Memorial Hospital, Donna Y., Dr. John Stock and a number of others, I was told to immediately get to the Women & Brigham's Hospital for Women located in Boston.

It was New Year's Eve, 1980, for heaven's sake! I was 23 years old. With a house party planned for the occasion, it was forfeited for my hospitalization. Packing an overnight bag with my husband driving, we arrived at the Boston hospital within hours. I honestly do not recall the midnight hour nor kissing him Happy New Year. I think he may have spent the hour alone, exhausted, after checking me in.

Chapter 13
Journaling day-by-day in black and white.

December 31, 1980

Making an immediate appointment at the Boston [Brigham and Women's] *Hospital for Women began with an ultra sound. This would apparently show how far along I was in this pregnancy and if I was eligible to use the "auto-syringes" and its program. This would then result with two days of blood tests to monitor my blood glucose levels with the constants of diet and insulin intakes. I like to think that the whole ordeal seems interesting enough to non-diabetics. However, it becomes tedious when a person, such as me, has been living as a diabetic for 21 years now. Well, my husband and I took this day-by-anxious-day.*

As clearly stated through the American Diabetes Association, "Diabetes, insulin treatment and high glucose levels are especially worrisome during pregnancy when they may jeopardize the health of both the baby and mother."

(Fund-raising letter dated October 24, 2005.)

Therefore, immediate placement in the Boston Brigham and Women's Hospital was adamant, elemental, and the only positive choice. To me this action meant that I had an actual chance, a hope, of birthing a child! That's what I wanted, what I needed. The support of my medical team would help me through this endeavor.

With it being New Year's Eve, my wish and main hope was for much wanted prosperity and good health for myself and this unborn child.

Cheers!

***

A. K. Buckroth

January 1, 1981.

Awakened at 3:30am in a cold sweat and shaking, I pressed the buzzer for the nurse. It's a low blood sugar reaction caused by too much insulin – hypoglycemia. These occur when insulin in the body lacks glucose to break down. Therefore, a glass of juice of any kind, as long as it has sugar in it, is a savior at a time like this. Soda or milk will suffice as well.

An hour later, 4:30am, more blood is drawn. As any diabetic can attest, the "drawing of blood" is constant, never mind being in this experimental pregnancy program.

7:00am was cause for a "fasting" blood sugar. These blood drawings, so to speak, are done with a finger stick device. When first a finger is chosen, it is then pricked by a small pin that will break the skin, causing a small trickle of blood. The blood is squeezed into a delicately thin glass tube for analysis. When fingers become sensitive or even calloused due to this daily procedure, ear lobes may suffice. I know and understand the procedures and their purposes. Never the less, they become very exhausting, even after just a few days.

I feel rushed, mentally, not used to this routine. There was no class or seminar on what to expect. Once the specialists learned I was pregnant – again – time was of the essence to save this embryo. I hoped the outcome of this tribulation is wholesome. When at home, I cared for myself with the "regular diabetic routine = diet, exercise and insulin injections." Clinitest tablets were once again used to test the urine for glucose content/control, thus the amount of insulin calculated on behalf of those test results. As mentioned earlier, the taking of blood is much more adequate and dependable. However, blood-taking devices – aka: glucose monitoring systems – were not readily available to me. Medical insurance coverage did not see this light. I forced myself to accept and understand that concept.

At one time during this hospitalization, I was allowed to leave for some fresh air. Even though that winter became known as the coldest since 1875, I just needed to get away from such a sterile atmosphere. I thanked my Higher Power for the coldness because it kept the bacteria away.

That district of Boston is nothing but hospitals! Being somewhat of a "healthy" patient, I was able to sign in and out as long as my wanderings didn't interfere with my inpatient schedule – that of having bloods drawn, scheduled meals and snacks, or other testing that may be required.

At 3:00pm every day, my husband got off work at the factory and made the 100 mile round trip to visit me. He insisted and I was grateful. He was my only "outside" visitor.

Wondering about this whole process, I seriously pondered if it was worth it. Afraid of the word "deformity," that was a high, factual risk with diabetic childbearing. Something I was not aware of until now. Everything depended on me, the mother-to-be. Strongly stated with any pregnancy, it became a warning, a threat, a frightful threat!

Yet all this seriousness left me a bit cocky. Past being bemused, a humorous sarcasm replaced the seriousness.

At this certain visit with my husband, we discussed what color to paint "the baby's room." Ooh, it was exciting to have been able to get this far, to actually be making a "plan." This discussion proved to me how hopeful we became since my admittance to this hospital. Everyone involved with my particular care was extremely supportive and encouraging. I never thought I would again be planning for another life. Biologically speaking, we had gone so far as to investigate the prospects of adoption. Presently on a waiting list in our hometown, that process took 3 – 5 years at the time. We even considered overseas adoption. Although an expensive and timely process, we remained on the list.

Back to the conversation, my preference for a room color was white-on-white with matching accessories and splashes of pastels. Although we discussed this before, it was still a tough subject. Being quite objective, my husband remarked on what we would do with the crayon marks when the kid got older! I had to laugh! This gave me positive food for thought.

146

Another midnight. Slumber approached slowly once again as my body and mind conjugate what is going on. I found myself pleasantly dreaming and anticipating the oncoming months. Never will I forget the past painful experiences. However, this is a whole new episode along with the whole New Year. Hopeful, I am constantly hopeful. Trying my best to be happy, not scared.

And it was just as well that I stayed awake! The "blood suckers" arrived for another testing.

As 4:00am rolled around, another low blood sugar reaction accompanied the time. This tells me that my evening insulin dose will have to be lowered. I neglected to mention that my diabetes has been controlled with two injections per day: one in the morning before breakfast, and the other in the evening, at approximately 9:00pm.

After that episode, I was awakened at 5:00am for a blood test and again at 7:00am for a fasting blood. Oh yes, there are the never-ending urine tests as well. There's no way of escaping this routine. My whole life has been consumed with this medical treatment. Being a juvenile diabetic, learning the processes for my care was imminent.

8:30am

"Well, you can start on the pump today," I was told. Hooray, hooray! Last night I was feeling not so energetic about this whole ordeal. The way I've been thinking is this: for one, the micro fine needle has to be removed daily, or even every other day, and filled with a solution of saline and Regular U-100 insulin. This is then drawn into a 100cc syringe. I'm just not exactly sure that going back to my normal daily routine would be just as efficient. Through the doctor's orders, regulations and whatnot, my "basal" insulin dose and a "normal" insulin dose are figured out and squirted through the tubing with the syringe hooked on one side of the machine. This basal regulation releases something like 1/10 of a unit of insulin every 8 minutes. I was started on twenty-two basal units. I have a remaining 24 units that will be dispersed a half-hour before each

meal and snack. After the total units of insulin are figured out and released into the tubing, the user (me) must calculate the basal and normal amounts by pressing a button and watching a small window where digital numbers are shown.

Sound confusing? Well it certainly is to me. But if fourteen women have done this before me already, and glad to do it, then so can I. The use and care of the machine is most confusing to learn at first. Oh yes, don't forget about the batteries! They're good for 24 hours and must be recharged over a period of 9 hours with the use of an adapter. All in all, with coaching and the enthusiasm from the attending nurses, I learned the routine in no time.

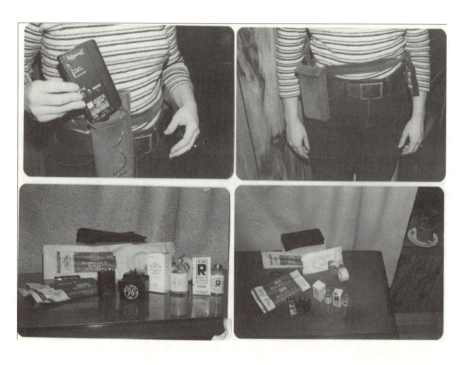

After all this is figured out, the micro fine needle is inserted below the skin on a 45-degree angle. It may be placed on any of the spots a diabetic customarily uses for daily injections. These may be upper thigh, arms, buttocks and lower abdomen. I chose the lower abdomen for insertion, as it seems to be the most convenient spot to enable movement most comfortably. I strap this mechanism onto one

hip and can move most freely. It may look a bit distorted, but so what if it's going to help me and my baby. So, I look like one hip is bigger than the other. That's certainly the least of my problems!

January 4, 1981

It certainly is amazing to see the hop, skip and jump effect of my blood sugars. A normal measure of sugar in the blood is anywhere from 80 to 120. And these are most important for regulation of my diabetes as well as that of the growing fetus. By amazing, I mean that a fasting blood sugar taken at 7:00am may be 80, whereas at 11:00am it could be 175, considering this is two hours after breakfast and a morning snack. In the afternoon, about 3:00, a blood sugar may have crawled up to 280; whereas at 8:00pm it has fallen back to 160. (This glucose measure varies per individual.)

As it was explained to me, this first trimester is the most confusing in getting the diabetic pregnant woman under normal and stable control as possible. As probably well known, with the growing fetus and your hormones doing somersaults, weird things happen to your body. It's a period of daily change and growth. I feel at this time that the diabetic, male or female, doesn't really know the extent of strict control of their disease until they've gone through a pregnancy. Self-discipline is so vitally important. One comes to really learn about the self and the problem! I am learning.

January 5, 1981

Oh heavens! I wanted to get out of this hospital! Any reader who has been in any hospital for any period of time can certainly understand my feelings!

1:00pm

That doctor must have been reading my mind! "Do you want to go home today?" asked Dr. Ryan, on e of the many attending physicians. No, actually I'd like to stay here for the rest of my life! Not showing any sarcasm, I was my ever polite and cheerful self saying, "Yes, of course, I'll get ready."

Well, after I was ready, I didn't realize I had to wait until my husband got home from work. And the wait lasted until 6:30pm. Boy, I was never so glad to see him!

8:00pm

Home. First thing I had to do was to set up this blood measure machine that was loaned to me through the courtesy of the Joslin Diabetes Foundation as well as the Boston Hospital for Women. I can at least relax for a few days until having to see any doctor. As they well informed me in the hospital, I must come to the pregnancy clinic at the Joslin Foundation every Tuesday for the next six weeks, or the duration I wear the pump, whichever came first.

After 10 days, I was equipped with an insulin pump and a glucose-meter detection machine.

Jeepers creepers.

Most of the stay there was due to the proper training and use of these machines. This was a first for me having to use both machines, never mind at the same time. [Little did I know that in the foreseeable future they would become my best friends, always by my side, literally!]

Well, we knew this whole ordeal wasn't going to be easy. An added 50-mile trip per week is worth the effort, worth a life! There was no guarantee concerning my health or that of my baby.

When I was told this, a heartless attitude seemed to strike me in the face. Optimism waned with reality. Blooming colors of hope began to dim. What an awful feeling.

We also knew the whole idea of the pump was experimental, but to know it and actually experience it are two different things. This is where I become very aggravated with the whole technique. Or, should I say, the diabetes research department.

Being diabetic for 22 years already, I anticipated a cure since early childhood. I recall, when at the approximate age of 8, there was a broadcast of a cure for 1971 - 72. Well, those years have come and gone, but not the hope. New techniques of fake pancreases and mechanical devices have since been spoken of widely. Yet this Auto-Syringe is to fare the end result. Yes, I am still disappointed, especially when the statement "we can't guarantee anything" is told to me.

I have personally blamed cancer and its research institutes for taking away the attention and monies that could have increased a cure for diabetes. This disease does not seem to get the attention it needs, especially in the public's eye. The onslaught of Aids at that time further ignited my anger, disappointment, jealousy, and frustration.

Please God, let them cure something!

Again, the dramatizations of hopeful possibilities through newspaper headlines have tried to enhance a sense of hope. For instance: *"Battle against diabetes continues while cure is sought;" "Drug shows promise in fighting type I diabetes" from the London Associated Press; "...supplement testing of diabetic children;" "Diabetes Alert: A Special Report; Miss America talks of life with diabetes;" "Treatments improve for Type 1 diabetics;" "Insulin offers better survival odds than pancreas transplant, study suggests;" "New insulin cell study may end injection need;"* and hundreds, maybe thousands of other articles covering decades. It is not that these headlines and journalistic artistry are steady, as in weekly or monthly updates. No, the articles come in spurts, more than a few at a time, at the same time, and relieve themselves never to be heard from for another couple months. This excited brevity causes interest in readership along with false hope. The public is becoming bored and non-caring. Like me, they have read it, lived with it, seen it, heard about it, etc., etc., etc.

Most recently, my mother once again wrote me "there is going to be a definite cure for diabetes this fall, 2006. They (some scientific researchers in Southern California), have found an injection of cells for the pancreas and has been FDA approved. This was on TV!" she announced.

Ah, ever so hopeful. I think it would be most beneficial for parents of diabetics to see that this was cured, never mind the diabetics themselves! As for me, I lost hope for myself. I think that the destructive progression that this disease is prone to along with my body's endurance of it for the past five decades will negate a cure.

However, I do look forward to knowing that the little ones are cured, the children. I do look forward to witnessing the day that a cure is available.

There was media coverage of still another device that could be implanted in the chest cavity of a worthy victim. But even so, they say that's a few years off. And how is a "worthy victim" determined? As I feel now, when a sure cure does come into focus, I may be too old. But let the here and now be a stepping-stone over deep waters. If what I am doing today will help solve a problem for such a confusing, baffling disease, let it be.

At this point in the pregnancy ballgame, my husband and I decided to keep this pregnancy a secret until definite, smooth sailing is underway. I'm used to secrets anyway. Surely you can understand why. People (especially relatives) get very excited about the oncoming birth of a new family member, a BABY. Through our past experiences, this may not happen, even now. Save the anguish of false hope. Now to conceal this curious "package" hanging on my side. I'll unbury some old "fat" sweaters and these should do the trick. I'm not one to save a lot of junk, including old clothes, but it's a good thing I hung on to these. Maybe I was anticipating getting fat - again. Been there too!

January 13, 1981
I didn't think I was going to enjoy Tuesdays at all for the next couple of weeks. First of all, it took me an hour and a half to get out there. Secondly, battling with those Bostonian drivers is like playing Russian roulette. Everyone on the road is an idiot but me!

One enjoyable reprieve is being able to visit my paternal step-grandmother, Nana. Her real name is Esther Underhill, but she will always be my Nana. She lives in Jamaica Plain, probably 10 miles from the Clinic, with Dziadzi (pronounced "ja-ji") which is Polish for Grandfather. His baptized name is John, and as step-dad to my father, we call him "dziadzi." He and Nana are the only grandparents we kids were to ever know. The biological pairs passed away long before we were born or shortly thereafter.

I fondly remember dziadzi driving to visit us kids and my mother a few times a year. He always brought us a bag of oranges. He had it in his mind that fresh oranges were good for me, being diabetic, and good for all of us in general their visits were never long enough. Dziadzi passed away years before when I was 18. He will always be missed.

I telephoned Nana to not only tell her the news, but to make sure I could stop by after my appointments. Delighted and cheerful as ever, she always had lunch prepared for us and made sure I got back on the road before 2:30pm when the traffic into Worcester starts getting bad each day. It is commuters' traffic.

Anyway, the doctor I dealt with today, a Dr. Burr, was extremely pleasant and took special time and care in explaining to me the procedures for keeping by blood sugars low and, therefore, under better control. "But doctor, I don't feel as good at an 80 count as I do at 150. I walk around with a persistent insulin headache and can't get anything accomplished. I also feel very drowsy."

"Andrea, the lower the better for you as well as the baby. There have been other patients with bloods as low as 50 or 60. The farther along in the pregnancy, you'll notice your bloods becoming very low, so be watchful of any reactions. At this stage, with so many changes taking place in your body, it is probably difficult to recognize a reaction. What you may have recognized before as a reaction can be totally reversed."

"So, in effect, what you're saying is that the signs I get now for too low sugar - sweating, shakes, hunger, drowsiness and whatever - may in fact be telling me that my blood sugar is too high."

"Yes, more or less. That's why we've supplied you with the blood sugar machine. Whenever you feel different - high or low - take a blood test to determine just where you are."

Oh boy, what an adventure this was turning out to be!

There was a simple pleasantry involved in these trips wherein I took advantage: my Nana Underhill lived in Jamaica Plains back then, so I decided to visit her every week after leaving these appointments. Over a prepared lunch on these Tuesdays, we tremendously enjoyed our time together. Having passed away in 1988, I miss her still, always will.

I continued to hope that all this aggravation is going to be worth it. You think this is confusing?! Well, dear reader, I am just as confused. After going over the week's blood sugar measures, it's determined that my basal dose (this is the one that keeps me regulated during the night and into the early morning hours) must be increased. Apparently, my fasting blood sugars were not satisfactory. Anyway, two units increased the dose.

In order to do this, a small screwdriver that came with the other paraphernalia, is inserted in the back of the pump. As I slowly turn the screw, I simultaneously press the digital read out meter button in order to determine the correct amount. Not very difficult. My basal measure is now at 24 units that are dispersed throughout a 24-hour period. The additional units stand at 8 pre-breakfast; two pre-morning snacks; six pre-lunch; two pre-afternoon snacks; eight pre-supper; and two pre-bedtime snacks. Thus, a total of 52 units of insulin are needed. This sounds like an awful lot to me, but, as the doctor also stated, "Wait until you get further along." I had always had the perception that the least amount of total units taken per day the better. Understanding that the more taken, the more of a strain one puts on the internal organs. Well, doctors' orders are doctors' orders. Ah, the life of a diabetic, a pregnant one!

January 15, 1981
Oh Lordy! What a fretful day this has been!
Keeping in order with my daily schedule, I awoke as usual at 7:30am to do the fasting blood sugar. No sooner did I get out of bed than I noticed that my nightgown was terribly wet. Oh my God! It was blood! Oh no, I can't go through this again. Oh God, no! I have to make it to the bathroom. I have to get a sanitary pad. Husband, call the husband. Oh dear God, back in the hospital again. He's got to take me to the hospital. He's going to miss work. Oh, not again. If this is another miscarriage I refuse to bear another child. He'll

understand. Thank goodness we started an adoption process already. What am I thinking? I don't know for sure. I'm still bleeding, but no clotting; small cramping. This is what happened before.

In between the hysterical weeping, I managed to call my husband at work. "I'll be right there, hon. Lay still until I get there. Call Boston and tell them we're coming in." He sounded as ill as I felt.

In the meantime, my blood sugar soared to a roaring high of 300 - fasting, no less. I took my eight-unit pre-breakfast dose and waited for my husband to get home.

Boston? Why the hell Boston?! I have an obstetrician in town. Well, they've been following me up until this point. Having called, I was told to be there as soon as possible. Well, as soon as possible took an hour and a half. In that time, I looked like death warmed over. And felt like it too! Upon getting to the Boston Hospital for Women, we had to wait for a while, of course. Why is that always the way when you go through such a catastrophic emergency or any emergency?

Well, my husband and I were both getting a bit agitated. I started crying again when the good doctor strolled in. After having checked me inside out, so to speak, I was told that I had stopped bleeding. And, if I were going to miscarry, there would be no way of stopping it. The big question was why did it happen? "We haven't an explanation of why or how," he said. "This happens to many women at this stage of their pregnancy. What we need now is to take an ultrasound to see if everything is all right in there. Since it is a holiday (Martin Luther King Day) that might be impossible."

After visiting with Dr. Michael Green, OBS, he did in fact verify that an ultrasound would be impossible. I'd have to stay overnight and wait until tomorrow. "NO WAY!" is what I'm thinking. Then I thought of a brilliant idea. Having asked the doctor to call my obstetrician, Dr. Karen Green, at the Memorial Hospital in Worcester, he did so without hesitation. He must have noticed my reluctance in being so far from home again.

After a few crossed wires and more waiting, he had gotten through and everything was all set. "If another emergency arises," he said, "don't bother coming all the way out here."

Now we were on our way to see Dr. Karen Green. Thank goodness. Did not think of her specialized care in that awful time of panic this morning. It was this Dr. Green that had first diagnosed me as pregnant and set me up with the specialized care in Brookline. She has also been with me through prior miscarriages.

Nonetheless, after many thank yous and whatnot, we suddenly got our appetites. Realizing that I had not eaten all morning, we stopped and had breakfast. Words between us were few as we concentrated on our own thoughts about the situation. We were most likely too afraid to say anything to the other in order to avoid hurt feelings. The truth always hurts.

Still looking like death warmed over, but feeling much more encouraged and "in the safe," we headed toward home - Worcester. I caught a few winks on the way, but still couldn't stop thinking about worse case scenarios. I held onto my husband's hand all the way home. The need for support was strongly felt between us.

Upon arriving at the Memorial Hospital and Dr. Karen Greene's office, we had still another wait. My spirit felt extremely numb at this point. I was mentally exhausted and wanted to fall asleep. Depression and anxiety took over my whole being. I looked like I felt - still. The doctor would know how to handle our doubts. We fully placed our trust and confidence in her.

After going over this morning's "rude awakening," she arranged for an ultrasound for 2:00 tomorrow afternoon. "Take it easy and get some rest until then. If anything more happens, especially the bleeding, don't hesitate to call." Don't worry doc, I won't.

The only reason I did not mind waiting for an ultrasound tomorrow was the fact that it was too late in the day to schedule one and I was home now. I felt more at ease since the Boston doctor restored our hopes.

January 16, 1981
Well, it wouldn't hurt to be there a bit earlier than scheduled. I'm

extremely anxious about this whole thing. After all, this will be the definite determination or not. I probably shouldn't have come as early as I did because there were quite a few people ahead of me. I also forgot about having to drink umpteen glasses of water in order for the ultrasound to work properly. This enables the bladder to enlarge thus putting pressure on the uterus to see the life inside. Interesting. I often wonder about modern medicine and its technologies. Some "inventions" are widely and properly used whereas others are kept hidden and secret. I mean, sometimes I have felt that if I were a millionaire (I should actually say trillionaire in this day and age) that certain other mechanisms would be used to obtain or keep my health in perspective. The medical world may be compared to that of a political one - the less you know the better.

After sitting in the waiting room thinking I was going to float away, I was lead into a fairly large, quiet room where this monstrosity of an ultrasound machine lay in waiting. It was hooked up, of course, to various television screens to show what was to be shown. Well, I couldn't make heads or tails of what was on that tube while the attendant scanned my belly with the "wand." She made it clear that I would have to get any and all information from the doctor. That meant more waiting.

January 17, 1981

It's a bright, sunny Saturday morning. Today is usually the day for housework and errands. Well, I'm taking it easy until I get a hold of the doctor. It was inevitable yesterday evening after the test. Another doctor was on call and couldn't supply us with any information. Anticipation. After all, Dr. Green has a family of her own to care for.

Let me tell you my mind was not in an optimistic viewpoint for the last couple of days now. I can't think of anything else. I keep going back to the last time I was pregnant and wondering if I'm walking around with a dead fetus. Oh God. It even hurts to think that, never mind say it. I seem to have separated myself from my husband for the time being. Don't like questions. It is a case of wallowing in self-

pity for a while. I am sure he is thinking of the same thing. We're both kind of numb in the brain and sick of thinking.

I finally got a hold of her a little bit after noon. She, as always, is quick to answer one of my calls. "Well, Andrea. There is fetal movement. Sorry it took so long to let you know. You and your husband must have been crazy with wonder. I've made an appointment for you in a few weeks. I'd like to see you before I go on vacation."

No kidding! I almost can't believe it! It's still alive! Oh boy, she doesn't know how good she made me - us - feel. Phew!

I would like to mention at this point that two of the nurses that work closely with pregnant diabetics, Barbara Gargnoli and Aimee Grause, have been in contact with me since I left the Boston Brigham and Women's Hospital. I actually feel that they're doing all the work: helping to regulate my insulin doses as compared with my blood sugars when I reported to them over the phone. Heavens, they've been in touch with me since day one, and always gratefully on hand when needed. In fact, I report with and to them first at the Pregnancy Clinic in Brookline before seeing any doctor. You would think that these two women were almost diabetic with all the close contact they have had with us "greenies." But they're not.

January 20, 1981

Another Tuesday. After the "traffic battle," I'm thoroughly un-encouraged and unenthusiastic about this whole trip. My attitude is deteriorating from the nonchalance it started with. I'm to see the teaching nurse today as well as the dietician, an obstetrician and a regular team doctor. Let's start with the dietician.

"Gaining weight awful fast, Andrea. What calorie diet are you on?" she asked.

"I'm on a 2000 calorie diet. I don't mind getting cut down a bit either. I noticed that I'm gaining too much weight and it's not baby fat. Don't want to overdo the blimp bit."

So, she cuts me down to 1800 calories, which is what I was on before I got pregnant. The increase came while in the hospital. Even with the strict exercise plan I put myself on, I'm still gaining weight at a fast rate. Heavens, I've been doing a total of 90 exercises so far that are increased by one every day. Also, I've signed up for swimming classes with a girlfriend and these are two evenings a week. That's especially tiring since I'm an occasional swimmer in the summertime. Plus, I walk three miles every other day. Believe me, I am trying to keep to this plan as much as possible. If I do get fatigued or too tired, I won't push myself. I already gave up on the spring and summer wardrobe, especially bathing suits. But, I'm not fond of this "fat feeling." Disappointingly enough, my Levi's don't fit anymore!

Now, onto seeing the OBS man at the Joslin Center. First of all, he went on to explain to me about volunteering for some type of breathing measurements. The whole process would measure my intake of carbon dioxide as I exhale. "We would be especially interested in you because of the pump," he went on to say. I felt he was trying to sell me something. And I asked, "Is this a step toward the cure or research of a cure for diabetes?"

"Well, no." he said. "It would just be interesting to find out and compare."

"Sorry, doctor, I don't mean to sound rude, but I don't see the point, or perhaps I don't understand what you're trying to accomplish. But I am not interested just the same."

When I want to, I can explain myself pretty strongly. He didn't like my answer. That was immediately obvious by the look on his face. Hoping to ease the situation, I asked, "Is there something else I could get involved in for the cure for diabetes. You, see, doctor, I have been a diabetic for almost 22 years, and at this point, a cure cannot be that inevitable." His generous reply was "Not unless you want to get involved with gene splicing." Well, not knowing what the heck that was and too afraid to ask, I repeated that I wasn't interested. Upon leaving the office he said, "Oh, I forgot to explain to you about your Hemoglobin A1C. Let's go back into the office." And I was hoping to get out of there early and save some money in the parking lot. Impossible.

My Diabetic Soul

With the door closed once again, he began with "Do you know what Hemoglobin A1C is?" Telling him "no," he went on to explain. "It's a measurement of blood taken over a period of the last four weeks to show your highest blood sugar count." Sounded like a sneaky way to do things, if you ask me. Anyway, he continued. "Your count this week was 8.6, which is fairly high." Interrupting him for a moment, I said, "But doctor, last week my count was 8.9 and I was told that that was great, yet I could be lower still." At this point, I was starting to feel very negative and agitated with this man. He went on: "Well, a normal pregnant woman has a level of between 4.0 and 6.0. Compared to this, yours is high. You may already know that the risk of deformities is higher than that of a normal woman compared to that of a diabetic. A non-diabetic has a 4% chance of bearing a deformed baby whereas a diabetic has between an 8% and a 9% chance. And it presently seems to me that you may have a 20% chance of bearing a deformed baby."

Well, I'll tell you! As soon as he said the word "deformed," I started crying uncontrollably. Yes, I've been forewarned about the statistics while hospitalized, but now it seemed like a threat "they" were hanging over my head. As any wounded animal would do, I started to fight back - with words. "Doctor", I began, "What you're telling me is that I could be already carrying a baby that could be born with missing limbs or eyes or kidneys or a liver?! Hey, I've been good, damn good!"

"Well, yes. Those are the possibilities. I'm just trying to tell you the facts. If I knew that this was going to get you this upset, I would have brought it up another time."

"Doctor, you're not helping me feel any better. And, frankly, I am not enjoying this conversation at all. All in all, you're also saying that if I have an extra piece of toast for breakfast, my baby is going to come out missing toes and/or fingers?!"

I the meantime, I'm balling my eyes out. What a scene. And there were no tissues in the darn office. In addition, this professional person sat there with me not even having the courtesy of offering me one. I went on. "So, the message I'm also getting is that I should think about terminating my pregnancy; about having an abortion."

His cool reply was, "That's up to you."

Well, I definitely had had enough of him for one morning. Making the excuse of running out of money to pay for parking, I got up and started leaving. He was alert enough to open the door for me. Gosh, I know my face was all red; I was still crying. I couldn't believe that conversation. Oh, I felt sick, I felt very sick. My head started splitting; I was angry and terrified. His demeanor was extremely questionable.

Upon arriving home, I calmed a ringing telephone. It just happened to be my Worcester doctors' secretary, Doreen, calling to tell me I have a urinary tract infection and that I'll be on ampicillin for ten days and how come I sounded so tired. Oh boy, all I needed to hear was her kind voice. Spilling the beans about my encounter this morning, she said she was definitely going to relay what I had just told her to Dr. Green.

No more than five minutes had passed when the doctor had called herself and wanted the story word for word all over again. She seemed very upset for me and thought that my blood pressure would be sky high. I informed her that I had the intentions of getting in touch with one of the Brookline nurses that was following my care. She said that I should, especially if that other doctor was telling this to other patients. I would get back to her.

Having called this particular nurse who had also seen me this morning, there was no answer at her number. I decided to nap for an hour, calm myself down, and try her number in an hour. My head was killing me.

5:15pm

Awakened by the ringing telephone, it was Aimee, the nurse. I explained as best I could about my morning encounters with this certain doctor. I could not even remember his name. Like an automatic mental block.

Aimee had said that my Hemoglobin was considered to be a bit high, but nothing to get overly upset about. That this certain doctor was highly exaggerating and she would tell another doctor about *this whole affair. Thanking her, I added that I did not want to see him in the clinic never mind have another appointment with him. I wanted nothing to do with him whatsoever. She guaranteed me this much and told me to get some rest and try to forget as much as possible about what had happened. I could do that.*

Come to find out some days later, through my Worcester obstetrician, the Brookline doctor had taken his numbers and facts from a pamphlet that consisted of facts and figures from a survey done a year ago using 100 women in one general area. Unbelievable. I had certainly better not see him again.

January 29, 1981

Feeling safe and comfortable, back in my own hometown, with my own doctor, today we had our first appointment.

The only thing I really dislike about being pregnant is the weight I've been gaining. Definitely no bikini this year!!

After the usual procedure of getting weighed and having my blood pressure checked, I was ushered into Dr. Green's office, gladly. She went on to check my belly, which at this point isn't very large at all. With the use of a compact machine and some type of jelly, she scanned my belly listening for a heartbeat. Ooh, needless to say I was absolutely thrilled by that sound. It goes so fast! I had no idea. If nothing else, that sound was most encouraging.

February 10, 1981

Back at the Joslin Clinic. I am wondering if they are going to take this pump from me today. I was given hopes of that idea last week when I had come for my usual appointment. It's now rather cumbersome. I have been wearing it everywhere including the shower, driving, etc. Not when I go swimming. And I quickly learned not to insert the micro fine needle into my thigh when wearing slacks. Ouch.

After the rigmarole of getting weighed (which I hate) and checking of vital signs along with the insulin dose, I was seen by one of the on-staff doctors. At the end of the usual fifteen-minute visit of seeing how I was doing, she asked me if I wouldn't mind departing with the Auto-Syringe machine. Well, in my mind, she really didn't have to ask me. Just take it! I knew I would have to give it up sooner or later anyway. I just wanted to get on with the inevitable reality.

This meant that I no longer had to travel to this clinic once a week. There exists a mixed emotion about that. So many nice people were involved in helping me maintain this pregnancy.

Trying not to appear rude or overly ambitious about getting rid of this new body part, I replied with a mild "sure." She went and put me on the usual insulin-syringe routine that I almost forgot about, if you can believe that. I knew eventually that I would have to go back to giving myself injections. I was spoiled using the Auto-Syringe.

Some of the nurses I had become acquainted with were on the scene to reclaim their "priceless treasure," or so it seemed. That Auto-Syringe was to be used, almost immediately, on another pregnant woman.

Yes, I was relieved and actually anxious to see how my usual manipulation of daily insulin doses would work out and further compare to this machine.

Departing with many thank yous and "I'll be in touch," I was warily sent over the Eye Clinic in another part of the building. Although the reasoning was not explained to me, I imagined that specialists wanted to see if any eye damage - retinopathy - existed at this time. Now that's a scary thought, but one that I have learned to live with throughout my life. Diabetes has lots of threats.

I was tested for glaucoma, which is oftentimes seen in the life course of a diabetic and known to cause blindness. In addition, cataracts were found with broken blood vessels (assimilation) behind both eyeballs. Good reasons to be frightened, pregnant or not.

Well, the examining doctor was astounded, to say the least. After going through all of whatever he had to do to find any problems, he exclaimed, "I can't believe this!" Hesitatingly I replied, "What is it you can't believe."

"Well," he answered, "let me ask you this. How long have you been diabetic? 22 years? How have you done it?! Your eyes are perfect. I cannot find anything - absolutely nothing - wrong. You must let us know your secret. I am going to display your pictures on the walls in the lobby."

Astounded much and myself relieved, I told him that I did not really have any secret, which I do not. Only my faith in God has helped me to feel like a miracle myself. And it's this faith that will help bring this child into the world in perfect health. Needless to say, I was very happy - ecstatic - to have heard that from such a renowned professional. I have good reason. A few diabetic friends have not been as fortunate as I. If not blinded through years of diabetes, some have died through other complications even though they were younger than I am now. And one thing I've dreaded among the many dreads is the deterioration of my eyes.

This has certainly turned out to be a fine day.

The eye doctor went on to tell me that he wants to see me just about every four to six weeks. This would prove helpful as I go farther along in the pregnancy. It is an ordinary precaution. And if that's the only time I have to come out to Brookline, well so be it. Now that I no longer have the machine, I am definitely resuming prenatal care in Worcester. If I run into any complications, I may certainly contact my doctor at the Joslin Clinic. Heavens, I've known him for fifteen years so far and am not going to cut off any ties at this point. Dr. Charles Graham and I met when I was eight years old. I was comforted to know that "they" at the clinic felt the same way.

In the next couple of weeks between February 10th and March 10th, I had definitely felt twinges of sorts along with sharp pangs and mild aches. The first thing one thinks of, at least I did, was that something was wrong. I knew this was not gas! Panic comes with any type of pain that shouldn't be. It took me a while to surmise what I was actually feeling was the child moving around. What a thrill that is! My doctor confirmed these feelings, which made my husband and I more excited. The aching in the abdomen is due to the muscles stretching, therefore allowing the child to grow and progress upward. I told myself that if that's all these aches and pains are, the more they are, the better we are. After all, you have to give yourself some redolent answers! Although my doubts for the both of us being healthy are becoming less and less as I expand, I still have many facts to weigh them up. And there's still the "if" factor. That will probably remain until this child is born. Only natural, right? If I sound paranoid, I am.

I would like to note that my insulin requirement dropped about 10 units as compared to the dosage with the use of the Auto-Syringe. As long as my blood sugars and urine test results remain level and low, there is no real cause for alarm.

March 12, 1981

Not only do I have to see a dietician today, but am also scheduled for an ultrasound this afternoon. I had asked for a meeting with a dietician because I seem to be gaining weight at an even faster pace. I was overweight once in my life and didn't like it then. Although my husband tells me I have a good excuse now.

Presently, I'm 4 months, 1 week, and 4 days along. And I've managed to gain 20 pounds. That's why I requested to see a dietician. I need some reassurance and a refreshing look at what I've been eating and how to put it under control - weight control. I would like my food intake put into grams so that I can measure each portion at each meal with the use of my trusty gram scale. Geez, that thing has been in a lower cabinet for years. My mother purchased it for me when I first began going to the Joslin Clinic many years ago. By using this, it would definitely insure the proper amount of calories as well as protein, carbohydrates, fats and the like. When one becomes pregnant, you can bet that your food intake will be watched closely, especially those of us who happen to be diabetic.

Upon meeting this dietician, who was quite young and thin as they usually are, we got down to the basic routine of what I have been eating daily so far, which would lead to what I do and do not need as of now. For instance, my daily dietary routine would go as *follows (taking into respect that all days are not the same and allowing for eating out):*

BREAKFAST:
1 whole English muffin with an 8 ounce glass of milk;
a 4- ounce glass of fruit juice, unsweetened;
one hard-boiled egg or a slice of cheese;
one cup of tea with two tea bags (I like strong tea).
LUNCH:
2 breads with 6 ounces of meat;
(i.e., a grilled cheese sandwich with four pieces of cheese);
8 ounces of milk and a small piece of fruit.
Along with this, I would make a small salad with no dressing or have a few carrots and celery sticks.
SUPPER:
I was required to eat 8 ounces of meat; the starch equivalent of two breads; 4 ounces of vegetables; the usual 8 ounces of milk, and again a small fruit.

As you may realize, this is an awful lot to eat, especially in the protein department. I neglected to mention that I was also required to have a mid-morning snack of crackers with 4 ounces of milk; an afternoon snack and an evening snack consisting of the same. Phew! Unknowingly at the time, the above listed to approximately 2300 calories per day. I thought I was on an 1800-calorie diet. No wonder I was gaining so much weight!

The following diet plan is what the dietician and I worked out before I left her office:

BREAKFAST:
8 ounces of low-fat milk; 2 fruits, which could consist of 1/3 cup of apple juice and a ½ grapefruit; or 3/4 cup of strawberries and a small orange;
2 slices of bread or 1 cup of cereal;
one meat portion, which would equal one medium sized egg or a slice of cheese.
LUNCH:

8 ounces of milk; 1 vegetable; 1 fruit exchange; 2 bread exchanges; 60 grams of meat (= 2 ounces) and 2 fats, depending on what you wanted in the way of exchanges which could be a 5-gram slab of margarine or butter or a teaspoon of mayonnaise.

SUPPER*:*

8 ounces of milk; 1 vegetable exchange; 1 fruit exchange; 2 bread exchanges; 120 grams of meat (= 4 ounces) and again 2 fat exchanges.

Having grown up with similar dietary plans along with the gram scale for measuring distinct quantities of food I know all too well what the exchanges are. What I find difficult at times is the problem of making up my mind to what I want. There is three of whatever offered and I can only have one or two.

For instance, as taught at Clara Barton Camp, one Oreo cookie OR two marshmallows OR one pack of "nabs," nicknamed for peanut butter crackers, was a snack. This is called "self-discipline" and it is very important. Otherwise I got terribly sick within two hours. Oh yes, there were times when I ate a whole roll of Oreos or half a bag of marshmallows, etcetera. An insulin injection of fast-acting "Regular" insulin was required in order to digest this junk. At the time, this Regular insulin didn't begin to work until half an hour had passed; I wasn't back to "normal" for another two hours, at least!

Though many of you may find this hard to understand, just remember that you cannot eat everything at once. And I'm sure your own physician would be more than helpful in explaining this further. Perhaps it would be a good idea to see an attending dietician to see how you and calorie intake go together.

Among the many pamphlets I was given, one that I found most interesting and helpful is the "EXCHANGE LIST for Meal Planning" put out by the American Diabetes Association, Inc., The American Dietetic Association, 1976. This lists quite simply and in detail all the allowances and exchanges one has to choose from in assuring that you not only get proper food requirements for your metabolism, but also the caloric intake.

All in all, this "new" diet brought me down to 2200 calories per day, which the dietician thought sufficient enough for my height, weight and the life of this unborn baby.

Not only did I leave her office with a handful of the usual pamphlets, but also with an air of accomplishment. I felt good about being good to myself. Having already started with drinking low-fat milk, I also encouraged myself to eat low-fat cheese, margarine and mayonnaise. You see, there are many ways you can work around getting fat - but that's just what it is - work and willpower. Oh, don't get me wrong. I cheated for sure. If I were to eat 2 English muffins for breakfast, I wouldn't allow myself to have any bread at lunch. Or, if I had two eggs instead of the required one, I would cut back on one of my other meals, always maintaining that certain caloric number during the day. I have to say again at this point that I feel lucky not to be having cravings. I would sure be in a lot of trouble if I did. My husband is dealing with that fact - and it's starting to show!

March 24, 1981

I am now wearing maternity clothes at 4 months. Can't hold it in or hide it any longer. I guess it's that "fat looking" stage that I've heard about. For a while I was just walking around without buttoning my pants and wearing a long sweater. But now I've given in, with my husband's insistence. I was tempted to try on his pants, but they look so big. Not that he's huge or anything, but an inch would probably be more comfortable. So, it's off to buy "prego" clothes. Not that I'm going to go overboard spending only because this won't last too long, or will it? And I can manage to sew some clothes that will help with the budget – especially toward the Baby budget!

Now everybody knows that I am pregnant. I cannot hide it. Some reactions were that of fear, knowing what I had gone through before. And still others were very excited and supportive. There are *those few that couldn't give a damn. I'm not sure how I exactly feel about this either. The medical entourage has taken so much of my personal thoughts during the beginning months. I realize now that I can really experience this as positive and nurturing. I should. I'm beginning to like this being pregnant. Healthy and happy.*

I think a woman goes through stages. I've already succumbed to the thought of giving up my body for the summer. I've also given up school, which was a big drawback for me. I'm now so close to getting my degree that missing another session wouldn't matter too much - or would it? Sacrifices.

April 9, 1981

Spring has definitely sprung, along with me. The ol' naval slightly protrudes from the belly. What an awkward sight. Quite ugly. If I happen to laugh or cough, it bounces out even more. Showing my husband is one sure way to get him laughing.

Today's visit with Dr. Green went well, as usual. She sees me every other week and I look forward to those visits. My due date is August 12th. My weight increased by three quarters of a pound each of these past two weeks. Normal, I'm told. Blood pressure - normal. And, every time I visit with her, I get to listen to the baby's heartbeat. Normal. I like that word – "normal, normal, normal." I depend on hearing that. It's reassurance for me that this child is alive and well. It makes me feel alive. I get frightened when the child is quiet - when I don't feel it moving around. It seems to prefer to remain in my lower abdomen and on the right side. This gets to be aggravating and uncomfortable at times. I think it's a foot that repeatedly gets caught in the right rib cage and I try to move it and rub it out of position. How absurd.

One time, I was consistently feeling twinges over a period of a few days. These twinges came every couple of seconds. When expressing my concern with Dr. Green, she laughed and said they were hiccups. Can you imagine?! Hiccups, of all things.

After having a light lunch, I was eager and excited about attending an ultrasound appointment. Yet there always lingers in my mind a doubt about the child being "whole" or growing at a slower rate than usual or even, in fact, that it had died suddenly. I was worried at the slight movements I feel, and when I do feel them. Perhaps I expected too much at this stage. I wanted to feel this child kicking and swimming around just to assure its mother that he or she was all right.

Again I found myself lying on a table watching a small television screen that doesn't display much, at least to me. I could not make heads or tails of what the attendant was looking for or finding. Suddenly she asked if I could see the head. "See, it is right there. And there are the eye sockets and an ear and the jaw bone." I was so excited I couldn't talk. Then she focused in on the whole body. The picture was more of a skeletal appearance where we could see a thighbone along with the calf, an arm and its fingers. One side of the head included an ear and a jawbone. The fetus was in a sideways position. What was most exciting was that we both witnessed the child slowly lift an arm and bend it at the elbow, flexed it fingers on that hand and proceeded to place its thumb in its mouth. "Can it suck its thumb already?" I asked. "Sure, they do all kinds of things," she replied. Then it took off as suddenly as it came. "Did you feel that?" the attendant asked. "No" I said. "Well, you've got quite a mover in there," she laughed.

Well, well, well. I was never more pleased, happy with myself. As I explained this to my husband, it suddenly occurred to me that as the fetus flexed its fingers before putting them in its mouth, the child seemed to wave hello. Hey, it's a nice thought. The friends and relatives got a kick out of it.

I can certainly say one thing - things are definitely shaping up positively.

Chapter 14
Thunder roars, lightning strikes!

July 20, 1981 at 5:00am, my water broke. What a frightening and embarrassing mess! I was home, lying in bed asleep beside my husband when I abruptly awoke, terrified! Was I was bleeding – again! After all, that has happened before!

"Hon, hon! Wake up! I'm all wet." I wailed through tears of fright. "Is this blood? The sheets are a mess. I can't look."

Groggily alarmed, he checked by touch. He didn't want to look either. "No, it's water. If you didn't pee the bed, your water just broke. Call Dr. Green."

Extremely big-bellied with pregnancy, I slowly, ever so slowly, lifted my legs over the side of the bed, and then lifted my belly in order to lift my body as a whole. Quite a maneuver! Through the bedroom doorway and into the kitchen, I telephoned the Emergency Room at The Memorial Hospital. I was told by the attendant/receptionist on the other end "to get a sample of the liquid, put it in a jar, and come in as soon as you can."

As I scurried to locate an empty jar, my husband had to call work. A perfect empty little jelly jar was kept in the laundry room purposefully for the storage of nails and screws. I grabbed it and scrambled to the toilet to do as advised. Sample in hand, we were out the door in minutes, arriving at the hospital at 5:30am.

Afraid to walk, a wheel chair was collected and I was rolled into the hospital. My husband went through the process of checking me in and met with doctors while I was rolled to the 2nd floor maternity ward.

Ahh, the time had finally arrived.

However, the wait was not over. During those seventeen hours of tiring and worrisome labor, unavoidable but expected discomfort also lead to other problems. The baby was breach with the umbilical cord around its neck and being upside down. Good Lord!!

After the infants' body was straightened out, grave decisions had to be made.

Well, the hell with what I learned in the few Lamas classes I attended! After three hours of having my knees atop my shoulders, enough was enough. There definitely is **no** dignity in giving birth! An epidural was ordered and given with the decision of a Caesarean section. Knowing in advance that this could be a possibility, my husband and I agreed to my having a Caesarean beforehand. Seventeen hours of labor is plenty long enough! Much to my heartbreaking disappointment, my beloved Dr. G. was unavailable. This baby was five weeks early and quite a surprise to everybody involved! No one was prepared. Isn't that the case with many newborns? I chuckle at the fact now.

The drama doesn't stop there!

Being wheeled into a delivery room, my husband behind my head with the surgical team in tow, I was prepped. I had my wits about me and requested the doctors to leave me with a 'bikini' scar. That was nicely done.

Awake during this birthing procedure, it just so happened that the anesthesia did not take full effect. I felt the slice. Having screamed and jolted with my upper body, the doctors quickly – and I mean quickly – resolved that situation! I felt the medication along with the necessary increase of numbness. For the next 18 months, as I healed from the C-section and did a new dance with life, that sliced area was more sensitive than painful. Phew! This experience became a definite factor with the long-term healing of my diabetic body. The efficiency and intricate care of my infant daughter and me was famously expounded!

As the surgeon was stapling the incision, one of the many nurses first brought the baby to my husband. "Hey, let me see my baby!" I screeched. The nurse briskly brought her to me and I could only touch her heal, quickly viewing her body for all the proper pieces.

She was fine as far as I could tell within those five seconds.

In the meantime, the attention to my blood sugar levels, blood pressure levels and all other body functions were taken care of continuously. I was then wheeled to a semi-private room.

My husband was sent home. He needed to rest. Anxious as I was to meet our daughter, the medical staff insisted I get some rest. I did. I napped. When my attending nurse finally brought her to me, I met my infant with elation through tears of joy. You can imagine! While I gently unwrapped her from her soft pink swaddling blanket, she fussed with tears and flexing her tiny hands. The nurse told me she was hungry. Well, I could fix that! Already having decided, and getting my doctors' approval to breast feed, the nurse helped me get her started. Such child/mother bonding is wordless. There was a deep sense of peace, a calming, a great respect and gratitude. I cherished every moment in gratitude for being able to go through this. I am wordless to say any more. I hoped and prayed that antibodies would pass on to this child. Think healthy, pray healthy, stay healthy.

Finally having decided on a girls' name, "Heather Dawn" was the end choice.

Due to the Caesarean procedure, Heather and I remained in the hospital for four days. Not only was I watchfully and meticulously stabilized, but Heather was diagnosed with a high bilirubin rate. From what I was told at that time, the highest rate was a 19 – she was there. I was also told that this is common through diabetic deliveries. I never ever heard of this being a factor; I never heard of *bilirubin* before this.

"She's jaundiced and has to be kept under the black light in an incubator. You'll only be able to visit her briefly."

Once told that fact by a chosen pediatrician, I burst out crying. I cried so hard I think I frightened the doctor! His face turned white, his eyes alight, and he became speechless. There was nothing he could do to console me. He sat across from me under the large hospital window, staring at me, and then abruptly rose to leave. A nurse arrived and spent more time with me, rubbing my back. No words passed between her and me.

My hospital roommate was gone, walking her newborn up and down the halls. I was thankful for the privacy. I was frightened. Thinking I did something wrong, nothing the doctor or nurses told me would calm my angst. I realize now that that crying jag was the "baby blues." It had to be. I did not experience anything close to that depression any time after Heather was born.

Before being sent home, the pediatrician visited me once again. As I was told by many of the nurses, he was quite thorough with watching Heather. Therefore, I was given specific instructions on how to help rid her of this bilirubin. She was to be seated in the sun, every day, throughout the day until we were to meet with him again in ten days for her first check up. Whenever she was brought to me for a feeding, I would sit in the hospital window with her, holding her up to the sun. I held her up to God through that window, introducing her to Him as if He didn't know. I thanked Him for this gift and vowed to take care of her with His help and the guidance of our Angels, Heather's and mine.

As we gloriously arrived home basking in all our "new parent" excitement, an unusual site greeted me at the driveway. It was an orange gladiola flower. But it was more than just a flower. You see, two years before this occasion I had planted numerous gladiola bulbs along the front driveway. Hoping that their beauty would greet friends, family and neighbors alike, they did not come to blooming fruition. I gave up, thinking that nothing would come from this planting. However, that precious day that we brought Heather home, lo and behold, there was a tall, lone orange colored gladiola. It stood there tall and happy in its greeting. I instantly knew what that was about, what that meant as soon as I saw it. It was a hello gift from the heavens. That is all I need to say about that. I believe. Through the years, I have continued to visualize that one lonesome flower as it stood tall and alone at the foot of our driveway. Another miracle!

It never bloomed again.

On the night Heather was born, a summer storm arose in the city. I recall seeing distant lightning flashes out the hospital window. Having been there for a total of seventeen hours, there was nothing more to do than try to lay still and glance at the picturesque storm. The later it got, the closer the storm came into the city. The sky was ablaze with white and yellow electrified lightning shards, roaring with sound, with booms and crashes! The accompanying rain drops dramatically and loudly pelted the hospital windows. For minutes at a time, this thunder storm took my mind off my pain before the epidural was decided upon. I couldn't help but notice that I later viewed this storm as a heavenly intervention, even perhaps, a greeting. The heavens, the universe, were releasing this infant in a blaze of glory! Another sign.

That first weekend she was home, friends and relatives were relentless in their visits. Although I was polite and courteous, I was exhausted and truly wanted them to leave us alone. I didn't appreciate people wanting to hold her, breathe on her, leaving germs. I didn't appreciate having to wait on them with coffee and tea. Heck, no one got the hint when I remained in a nightgown for two (or was it three?) days. Being out of the hospital I hadn't checked my urine sugar. I ignored myself and it seems that everyone followed suit. I couldn't bathe because of the staples. I couldn't, and wasn't supposed to, stand for very long and the fatigue washed over me.

My husband was at work meaning I was home alone with the infant. I only ate well because I knew Heather needed nourishment and that came from me. It didn't take long – ten days to be exact – that I was back in the hospital for another ten days.

"Andrea, wake up," my husband was yelling. "Wake up. You're shaking and twitching. What's wrong?! Do you want to go to the hospital?"

"Yep," I replied. "Call Dr. G. Tell her what's going on. I'll get me and the baby dressed." I had had a convulsion. Surprise, surprise! Not too good when I have 36 staples in my gut!

"No, we're not taking Heather," he said. I'll call Janice and see if she can take her."

Well, neighbor Janice was able to take Heather and keep her during my hospital stay. What a fiasco that was! Because I was breastfeeding and insisted on doing so, my husband woke up extra early before having to go to work. He came to the hospital to collect my breast milk each morning, and brought it back to Janice for her to feed Heather each and every day of those ten days. Then he had to go to work which lasted until 3:00pm or 3:30 each day. After work, he would clean up as usual, collect Heather from Janice and bring her up to me. He was so exhausted. The exhaustion and fatigue were set in his face. On more than one visitation, he fell asleep on my hospital bed. I didn't disturb him. My family was here: my husband, asleep, and my baby safe in my arms. Little blessings.

While he slept, I was able to leave the hospital room and gingerly pace the halls with Heather in my arms. We became acquainted, she and I. As soon as a nurse chastised me for being on my feet, I would return to my room, cradling my infant. Heather's father was awakened by the nurses each night because visiting hours were over. Those visiting hours were repeatedly extended. The nurses were informed of what was going on. They knew. Small kindnesses were granted and greatly appreciated.

Once awake, he would gather Heather, tuck her in her car seat, kiss me goodbye, go home, and then start the next day over again with the same conditions.

Not many visitors came to see me. To this day, I think people were afraid to get physically close to me thinking they would spread germs and make me worse. They didn't want to be involved in this expansive drama. After all, it was the initial hullabaloo that got me into this trouble. However, my very best friend at the time, Denise B., showed up briefly, whispering in conversation.

"You don't have to whisper," I told her. "We're out of danger."

"Are you sure?" she asked. "The nurses told me to be very quiet."

"I'm out of hot water right now and intend on staying that way. This was a fluke," I replied and explained to her. Gosh, I was so happy to see her!

Denise brought baby gifts galore too! Gifts are always fun. But she explained to me that "this weekend I was having a baby shower for you. With the baby's early arrival, it was canceled. And now that you're feeling better, people will be allowed to come see you and leave the baby gifts."

Ah, I was disappointed. I love parties, especially when they're for me. Oh well.

She did let it be known that it was safe for others to come visit me. And they did. Gosh, after being practically isolated for five days, I was starting to get depressed. Happiness is grown when shared.

At one time during this emergency hospital stay, one of the two birthing surgeon-delivery physicians came to visit me. He was alarmed that he didn't find me in my bed with my infant. I was in the restroom, sitting on the cool floor, breastfeeding. It was an extremely hot and humid early August day, there was no air conditioning, and people were allowed to smoke cigarettes. So, I did what I believed was the right thing to do for Heather and I. I took her out of the smoky atmosphere, away from any person for privacy purposes, sat on the cool tiled floor against a cooler tiled wall, and fed her.

The look on his face when he opened the restroom door and found us was one of complete surprise and shock. I can visualize it now. He could see what I was doing but I had to explain my rationale. He agreed. Helping me back to bed, he closed the main corridor door and commenced a conversation about my improved health. For the life of me, I cannot remember his name. I remember a young, handsome face and body, but no name. My regret.

"You're doing much better and will be able to go home," he said. "However, you have to take it easy," he continued sternly.

"Okay, okay, I will," I said, really saying anything to be able to go home. Ah, isn't that what a sick person longs to hear? I could have screamed of happiness!

"You no longer have a fever," he continued "There is no infection.

You should be back in a few weeks' time to have the staples taken out."

I do not recall the rest of the details with their instructions. I knew what I had to do. And I wanted to go home!

For the first two and a half years of Heather's life, I was a stay-at-home-mom. This period of time greatly helped me heal, recuperate, recover from the last three dramatic years. I greatly enjoyed being a mom. With her daddy having to work every day and every night because he got a second job, Heather and I shared nothing but time. In the summer we walked downtown quite often. That was approximately a 10 mile round trip excursion that happened at least once a week. She was seated in a stroller of course, which I believe is to blame for her current scoliosis.

Heather and I occasioned a matinee, with her first ever movie being "E. T." We drove to the ocean, where I was anxious to introduce her to that part of nature. There was always a park to visit or a toy to ride or a game to play in the yard or driveway. We cooked her daddy's supper every night and visited with Grandma Ruth and Poppa Edwin. Her paternal aunts and uncles were an occasional factor.

The New England change of seasons always brought a weathered gift of one sort or another. Enter autumn with Halloween when I made her first Halloween costume. Snowy winters brought out snowsuits, sleds, ice skates and building snowmen. I stayed active with her. I was obsessed with giving her most of my attention with love. I didn't know if I was going to live long enough to plan for a future with her, if she would end up being left motherless because of my diabetes. I needed to see and experience everything I possibly could with Heather while I could, one day at a time.

This zeal for life was not appreciated or agreed upon by my husband. I had places I wanted to go, people I wanted to meet and many things I wanted to accomplish. He wanted me to go back to work fulltime, in a factory. There was no encouragement for life, for further education. He did not share my zeal. My passions were intangible. He was a Union factory machinist worker, was raised by factory workers. His was a hard life. What I consider a poor attitude on his part was reflected with his family. Eventually, I learned what it was to be an "outlaw" as opposed to an in-law.

After too many denials toward my expansive potential and empowerment, especially those that required his financial support, I left him. Support of any kind was not present. Financially, emotionally, sexually, spiritually, etc. My yearning was not understood or appreciated. Therefore, I took Heather and left, leaving him with the home we made, with the house we bought using my grandfather's inheritance money.

Now I was a single mom. I never ever regretted a day of that role. When I look back at this transition, it seems I repeated history, having been brought up by a single mother. I knew this gig.

That entire marital honeymoon hubbub with the miscarriages, the abortion, and the adjustments involved with an infant with my health being at stake, I realized I was not appreciated as a human being striving to stay alive on a daily basis. I was not encouraged but held back. This relationship lasted a meager five years before I realized that it was not healthy. I released myself from a type of bondage; uncomfortable and unshared feelings were let go. The divorce was final on February 14, 1983. The irony was a gloomy Valentine's Day.

Chapter 15
Freedom-again!

Having found an immediate secretarial/receptionist job in a nearby computer retail store, I was able to settle into an apartment close to Heathers' preschool. We began a new life together. With the monetary amount in the divorce settlement along with household furnishings, and a 1981 Chevy pickup truck, I was able to set us up comfortably. The largest expenses were for a refrigerator, a stove, and parlor heater. It took a little time, but it all got done.

Before my engagement and consequential marriage in 1978, my college studies were well on their way. I was encouraged to contact the Massachusetts Rehabilitation Foundation for financial assistance. After qualifying with this organization as well as receiving a government Pell Grant for my tuition, my college courses along with every other expense – books, pads of paper, pencils, etc. – were completely paid for. After marriage, I lost my qualification. Life went on. Struggles ensued.

In June of 1984, I was finally able to graduate Quinsigamond Community College with an Associate in Science Degree. Hurrah. This endeavor took me nine years. Nine years to accomplish a two-year degree. Well, it's over now. An accomplished struggle was what it was. No regrets. I denote my selling of Avon Products for assistance in this endeavor.

My zest for knowledge continued on to Worcester State College. Wanting to gain a Baccalaureate Degree in Business Administration, I chose AFDC (Aid to Families with Dependent Children – Welfare) to assist in this endeavor. It was the only way to accomplish this goal as a full-time student, graduation expected in five years with the course program I chose. Having been laid-off again, the decision was easy. Go to school. Once again, classes and supplies were covered. However, the monthly financial allotment that was supplied personally kept me in the poorhouse.

Medically covered under the State's Medi-Care benefit, our health expenses, my persistent supplies, along with heat and gas were covered. Allotted $402.00 per month with $85.00 in food stamps and $50.00 per month in child support, making ends meet was hair splitting. This lasted five years until I graduated. $400.00 a month went for rent. Once a month grocery shopping consisted of macaroni & cheese, usually 4 for $1.00; frozen bags of vegetables; hot dogs; chicken thighs; a splurge with ground beef; flour, sweetener; and a few pieces of fresh fruit. If anyone I knew had a fruit tree, it was sure that I would be over to pick some fresh fruit for us. It was the same with anyone who had a vegetable garden. There were no extravagances. Being diabetic is not cheap in more ways than one, most especially when dietary necessities are hard to come by.

I never understood how the State of Massachusetts was able to demand and collect $85.00 a week from my ex-husband and gave us $50.00 a month. It doesn't seem fair. Afraid to ask my social worker any questions, I kept my mouth shut and humbly kept on.

Heather's school dress code, after kindergarten, required a uniform. Before that, her grandparents bought her some of the cutest clothes. Being born in late July, birthday presents always consisted of new shoes and jackets along with a new wardrobe. My mother was adamant about buying Heather's shoes at Stride-Rite, a professional shoe retailer. With Christmas just six months away, the gifts were repeated. I feel blessed by God, again, in that respect.

To assist us in this lack-of-money-situation, I established a typing business out of our apartment. Through the extra attention given to me from a former College Professor, my typing skills greatly improved and gave me a great sense of self-confidence. I could do this!

Supplied with a Commodore 64 computer and printer from my sister, Judy, I was now able to print advertising flyers. These were tacked onto kiosks through the eleven colleges in Worcester. With a rate of .50 (yes, 50 cents per page) with a 24-hour turn-out time, I was able to gain a separate yet scant income. This greatly helped to supplant our better eating and provided gas in my truck. My typing capabilities were a superb talent and included correct punctuation, sentence structure, spelling, and grammar. Most of my clients were young college men. At that time, typing was still a girls' job. I was often amazed at the incomprehensible and hand-written documents many of these students wanted me to transform for them. Being a college student myself, I was very familiar with professorial expectations. I had to do something to get us fed properly!

Single parenthood is a challenge. Health and finances were two of my biggest tribulations. Already familiar with sacrifices, this adjustment brought challenges disguised as sacrifices and vice versa.

Before being laid-off from the second Administrative Assistant position where I worked for 2½ years, Heather and I were able to visit Europe. I made a promise to my grandfather, my dziadzi that I would do this and I did. Paid vacation time and a small savings account granted this dream. Most of this two-week vacation time was spent in Germany. A U. S. Army Captain friend of mine (last known as "Major" Robert McElroy) from high school had lent us his apartment. After Heather recovered from a three-day virus, we were able to adventure to our heart's content. I do admit that this adventure maxed out my credit limit, but it was worth it! Having taught myself the German language with library LP albums and books to include the English – German dictionary, train rides, restaurants, boutiques, markets, and small general conversation was pleasantly and proudly accomplished. We leisurely traveled through France and visited Luxembourg which I absolutely fell in love with. Heather, being three years old at the time, became ecstatically excited with the trains we rode every day as well as with the mansions we visited. She ate and slept well – we both did.

The early '80's was a great learning time for me professionally and personally.

To further deal with expenses, I joined a "Powder Puff Mechanics Course" at a local high school in Worcester, Massachusetts. The class was once a week for twelve weeks. This was one of the best decisions I ever made.

Having repeatedly invested in repairs of my 1981 Chevrolet Cheyenne pick-up truck (5-speed on the floor) with no satisfaction, I was determined to take care of it myself. My sister, Gina, once again baby-sat for Heather while I attended these night courses.

As I was the only woman in attendance, I suspected that the other students thought I was a lesbian. None of 'those guys' ever spoke to me or simply greeted me. It was a 'guy thing,' a 'guy club.' So be it. Even the teacher didn't waiver with his manliness due to my presence. I did not intimidate him. That's a good thing. I was there to learn. I was a good student. I needed to learn about how to take care of my truck and any other vehicle I came across. This truck was a big part of my life, our lives.

In a way, I became a man. I see myself as having dropped my feminine exterior not only to wear the required mechanics' jumpsuit, but in other respects. I became tougher, more calloused, able to lift a tire out of a trunk, change a set of spark plugs, check all of an automobiles' fluids, change its hoses, swing a wrench, install a battery, install a radiator, keep it clean under the hood, and more. I was silent. I didn't boast about what I was doing. However, I was proud. My mother was in awe. And my fingernails were dirty. I grew into a new self-comfort of independent pride.

During this 12-week course, I was adamant about my medication. There was no way I would allow myself to have an insulin reaction, to have to drink juice or eat sugar. There was no way I was going to admit to being weak in any way, shape or form! I was not going to embarrass myself! My strategy worked. My strength of body and mind worked well together to accomplish this goal. I was empowered through strategic planning without even knowing it!

The ease of working on and in this pick-up truck was phenomenally easy compared to the computerization of vehicles these days. Years later, in the late '90's, I took another course in a local high school in San Pedro, California. Eight hours every Saturday was one requirement for five months. It was awful! I was not the only woman this time, but I was the only 'white woman.' The Hispanic teacher insisted on speaking Spanish with the majority of students. Another student, a young Caucasian male, and I, briefly befriended each other if only due to being able to speak fluent English – to each other!

My purpose to take this specific course was to learn how to handle the computerized auto mechanics. What I learned was what I already knew. It was disappointing and I never stayed to finish and get my paper certification. I was, and remain, disappointed after all these years.

The diabetes remained in check. Lunches were not supplied, so I brought a lunch to every Saturday's class. At this time I had a 1984 Volvo DL242. I sat in my car and ate my lunch. That was nothing new to me. It was better than having to hide and eat in a restroom! Not only was I discriminated against, but I purposefully stayed away from the majority of other students. We couldn't communicate verbally! My four years of high school and college Spanish courses were insufficient.

All in all, the knowledge I gained has remained thoroughly useful. Not only have I diagnosed problems with my own vehicles, but problems in friends and acquaintances, and their friends and acquaintances as well. However, there is always a man to get in my way and try to shut me down, disapprove of my diagnoses until he gets it proven. I've been right, many, many times. But, I've never heard it from a man: "You were right about my car." Never. I'm just supposed to stand there and look pretty. Hah!

Too many times my mind has reeled in anger. The arrogant and smug male is counterproductive to my quality of life. I always did and continue to keep my mouth shut in the company of a man when discussing formerly and supposed "masculine" projects (e.g., autos, tools, wood works, driving, water heaters, plumbing, etc.) I despise being under-estimated. It's not worth it to me to argue my knowledge, my worth. I agree such an action is disrespectful, but I avoid arguments in that way. Arguments make me physically sick, and I can't and won't afford that. I shut up. I'm alone in myself. I am comfortable there and familiar.

Yes, I've also taken a course on plumbing.

With a newly acquired business degree, the career I fell into was one secretarial/administrative job after another. Due to the formerly mentioned computer store having closed, my résumé grew from this experience. Through the store closure, another adjustment was at hand = looking for another job.

Dating again was fun but awkward at first. I really had no interest in anything but Heather and my futures. That changed once I got into a groove of knowing what needed to be done and doing it. The universe knows I've known enough men, had enough lovers that the sex was not unfamiliar to me. It was the hypoglycemic reactions after or during sex that brought me panic. It was a lover that was not familiar with them. Unless a solid commitment was coming on, I never told him I was diabetic. There were not too many men that I spent time with that kept orange juice in their refrigerators or any type of quick acting ingestible stabilizer to erase the symptoms, to normalize my body. Conclusively, bachelors eat out – a lot, all the time! I would have to scrounge through my pocketbook for sugar packets. Knowing that I needed to eat 20 – 30 minutes after a hypoglycemic episode, breakfast or lunch was a perfect persuasion. In the meantime, I resolved to keep snack food (e. g., peanut butter or cheese crackers, small bags of peanuts, along with Glucose Tabs) with me at all times, in my pocket book, purse, brief case, and the truck door pockets. This habit of keeping snack food available continues to this day and has come in handy for not only me, but other adults and children that are in my company and automobile.

Flying had been a wished for accomplishment for a long time. I truly wanted to have a pilot's license, to gain that knowledge along with the knowledge of the mechanics of an airplane. I do not know where my initial inspiration came from. I wouldn't call it a dream. If I wasn't diabetic, it would have been a dream. It was a thought. A temptation.

Through and because of a required thesis for a class at Worcester State College, I chose to research and write about the future of corporate flying. I wrote about the efficiently of such a task as opposed to other vehicles that were, and remain, in use. That paper began with the history of flight, its present and daily use at the time in 1988, ending with a premonition of over-crowded flies-in-the-skies.

This project so endeared a quiet yearning for me to accomplish, that I inquired as to how, what, when, where, and how much it would take to start, and finish, with a private pilot's license. I was not interested in flying commercially!

Well, I was rejected by immediately told "no" due to "the imbalances of diabetes." Our conversation implied that the obtaining of such a license "would be a great liability and not worth the time and effort." And my having to wear glasses was a stipulation as well. I didn't fight it. There was only that one person that I spoke with, purposely as an interview for this college thesis. But I was curious just the same. I didn't fight it because there was a grain of truth in what I was told. Through my own experiences, low blood sugars and high blood sugars are an uncomfortable constant, making me temperamental and occasionally physically ill. The FAA (United States Federal Aviation Administration) has strict medical requirements. I didn't want to have to go through that bureaucracy. The other stipulation to this dream was the expense.

During my aforementioned marathon training I met a young man, Ron S., a diabetic pilot. I was overwhelmingly amazed and enthralled, delighted, prideful, and jealous all at the same time. He went through the required rigmarole and flew Cessnas and Pipers.

Then I read about a guy out of Scotland, Doug Cairns, also a Type 1 diabetic, who flew around the world! Oh my GOSH!

And that's not the end of it!

A. K. Buckroth

While attending a "California Capital Airshow" in March of 2006, I met diabetic pilot Michael Hunter! He was promoting "Flight for Diabetes: a not-for-profit organization with 100 percent of proceeds benefiting children with diabetes." My attention was first grabbed by the advertisement of 'Accu-Chek' on the side of his plane. Accu-Chek is one of the many glucometers (blood sugar testing device) in use by diabetics. There was also another advertisement that read "Flight for Diabetes." Boy was I delightedly surprised! He wore the same type of insulin pump I do and we briefly discussed the pumps' flexible efficiency! He "has made history as the only diabetic person in the world with an FAA low-altitude air show license" as he performed at the show in his Laser-230 monoplane.

It wasn't until meeting Michael that I learned, from him, that the FAA "changed its policy due to the advances in diabetes control." That is how Ron was able to accomplish this feat. I just didn't know or was too busy with my life in 1997 to pay attention.

Well, with all this delightful news, I do not regret pursuing and attaining that dream. My accomplishments were steered elsewhere. I passed my flying dream onto my daughter, who began instruction at Torrance Airport, California, at the age of ten.

Employment opportunities were not as bountiful as hoped. Scoping the main Worcester area newspaper, certain agencies were continually listed and hiring people with my skills: typing, filing, dictation, telephone messaging, vendor greeting, etc., the typical secretarial duties. I was able to give more. With two business degrees to boot from Worcester colleges, my empowerment was piqued. The required wardrobe – business attire – was graciously and gratefully maintained through neighborhood thrift stores. With my amiable personality, full-figure, a pair of legs that wouldn't quit, who would not want to hire me. Remember, I take care of myself. I not only have to but I want to – I want to live a productive life! And I can put on the charm as well as another.

Come to find out in this job search, Temporary Agencies are numerous. With that being said, I applied to 17 at one time, in order to land myself some work. Part of the application process requires an applicant, me, to perform a typing test for speed and accuracy, the use of computer software proving computer literacy, a math test, and a generalized personality and appearance review in order to be placed in the proper organization. I was required to call each agency on a daily basis to inform them that I was or was not available.

The "temporary" work was a wonderful opportunity for me. Not only was I able to use my brain to accomplish what needed to be done in any organization, but this allowed me time to schedule necessary and various types of doctors' (endocrinologist, chiropractor, dentists, dermatologist, gynecologist, orthopedists, ophthalmologists, optometrists, neurologists, pediatrician, etc.) appointments for myself and my daughter. I had the responsibility of filling-in for Administrative Assistants due to their vacations, firings, and/or maternity leaves. The longest time I was ever at one place was 9 months.

Although many of these work environments were conducive to my overall monetary benefit, there were a few that were not. To begin with, I quickly learned not to tell an interviewer that I am diabetic. The few times I did, I never heard from him or her. When I did choose to disclose this personal information, I purposely did so for the welfare of those I would be working with. Rationalizing that decision was due to my concern about people I didn't even know, never met, but would possibly work with. Is that stupid?! My thought process was that if I ever went into a convulsion or couldn't help myself as happens when a person loses consciousness, someone would know to not only call for emergency assistance but report that I am a diabetic. Wouldn't they? I don't know. I never gave anyone the chance. I couldn't and didn't trust anyone but myself. "I am not drunk, I am diabetic."

One particular job I took was for a receptionist position in a mental health facility. I was to operate the front desk, alone. The office manager, a heavy set, unkempt woman of 50 years old made it clear to me about my not only leaving the area to use the restroom, but had a strict policy of no eating at the front desk. I could appreciate her concern and respected the regulations. I had to. I need this job. I needed the money. After all, patients were coming and going and needed to be greeted and assisted properly. "Properly" meaning no food in your mouth and no being seen sipping a beverage of any sort. I was to be robotic, inhuman. When I needed to use the restroom, I was to buzz this specific office manager who was supposed to sit in my place until I returned. Unpleasant as she was, it took her 20 – 30 minutes to relieve me and she yelled at me for taking 4 minutes to pee! One of the physicians happened to witness this verbal abuse and took her aside. He wanted to know why I didn't have water to sip on at my work station and got me a cup of water. Humiliation put aside, I was busy contacting my temporary offices for another position, having to explain to them my restroom story.

That wasn't the worst of it. I have many such abusive stories, with slightly different details.

For example, at the time of holding this position and for many, many years before, my diet required a morning and afternoon snack, approximately 10:00 am and 3:00pm respectively. This typically consisted of peanut butter crackers, or 2 graham crackers, or 15 grapes – something that I could consume in an unnoticed hurry. I preferred not to overextend this time frame by more than 30 minutes. However, what I wanted and needed didn't always come to fruition.

The only place I could eat my snacks was in the restroom. Uncomfortable and illogical to me, I had to do what I had to do. Nobody knew, once again. Nobody knew because I concealed most everything – snacks, sugar packets, medication. I repeatedly avoided any possible confrontations about my disease, in turn avoiding potential problems. I kept it a secret. Oh my gosh! Forget it if I needed juice or a quick 'sugar load' because of an insulin reaction. Due to a co-worker taking too long at their lunch, or my having to work two stations because of an unexpected 'no show,' my scheduled breaks often became non-existent. Begging to go to the restroom so someone would relieve me, I'd scurry there to eat something the fastest way I knew how. It wasn't good. Upon my return, negativity abounded with a chastisement, or a demanding degradation. Because I was a "temp," did this mean I was to be abused or disrespected while being used? The only reason I put up with it was because of money.

This frightening game I played was meticulous and manipulative to the 'enth' degree. If I felt hyperglycemic and needed insulin, I would somehow manipulate a co-worker to cover for me and give myself an injection. Doing this takes time. There are no shelves in restroom stalls in order to rest anything upon, such as an insulin kit. The floor had to be used. Undressing and doing my business takes long enough without having to roll a bottle of insulin, uncap a syringe, measure the units needed, squirt out the air bubbles, and then inject.

"What are you doing in there?" a co-worker would ask as she heard unfamiliar sounds in my stall. These 'sounds' were my rolling the insulin bottle between ringed fingers or the sound of opening and closing of my plastic insulin case on a tiled floor. Strange. I did not make 'noise,' per se, but 'sounds' that some co-workers thought unusual because they were!

"What took you so long?" I would hear when I finally got back to my work area. I usually blamed the use of time on 'getting my period 'or seeing'Mr. So-And-So in the hall' or stopping at the bubbler for a sip of water. I didn't doddle, purposely. These inquiring souls just didn't want to be where I was supposed to be and thoughtlessness overcame kindness. Time and time again.

There was more than one occasion, at different work sites, when I could swear – but not prove – that I was being watched, even having been followed. You see, being "a temp" has a degree of mistrust for those whom I worked for and with. I wasn't really "one of them," a naturally hired employee but "a useful conduit to get jobs done." That fact in itself never seemed to be appreciated. Uncomfortable as the truth maybe, I was used for another's gain. The irony here is that I was paid for my knowledgeable submission.

I'm happy to admit that I've never passed out or had to be rushed to the hospital from any of the innumerable work places I encountered. I maintained personal control, physically, mentally and psychologically. It's tiring!

I would like to know that diabetics can take proper care of themselves in the workplace. I would like to know that a diabetic can inject his or her medication when needed, with ease and comfort. Not necessarily out in the open, sitting in an office cubicle chair. Use of discretion is required! But having to hide the fact that it is something that needs to be done is unacceptable, unthinkable. Respect the fact that controlling this disease is a matter of life and death through minute details! Some people have forgotten the meaning of the word "respect," especially respect for others. "Consideration" would be another prime factor.

Chapter 16
Traveling and overnight scenarios.

Ahh. Being a career can girl carry many positives things with it: independence, financial pride, self-pride, confidence and self-worth. At least it did for me. My optimism never failed; it may fade at times, but it always resurfaces.

Socializing was fun, dancing every weekend, being wanted and needed by friends just for my company, insight, or conversation. I was my own woman, a self-made woman. I liked me. Still do.

Once financially stable, I was able to invest in some beautiful suits, out fits, coats and shoes. I was able to travel with my daughter, visiting Europe one year, Canada another, Oahu, and Florida. Of course, we conquered the close and various New England states with their majestic views and sea coasts; dining on steamers, lobsters, fried clams (one of Heather's favorites), and/or clam cakes.

Most of the travels with my daughter involved my driving except to Europe and Hawaii, of course. A cooler was packed with lunch meats, a loaf of bread, milk, juice, water, carrots, celery, fresh fruits and my insulin pack. I was always conscious of the need to eat and to eat properly. My daughter, so very young, was extremely aware of this and took it as being normal. When most folks would stop to eat at fast-food places along any number of highways, we stopped at rest stops to use the facilities and picnic with our own goodies. She witnessed on numerous occasions my having to inject insulin while sitting behind the steering wheel. The most convenient spots were, and are, my lower abdomen or upper thigh.

Traveling. Hmm.

While still at home, my mother's house, taking that alcohol filled metal container with its glass syringe and metal needle was commonplace when we traveled as a family. We never stayed overnight. Remember, this was long before disposable syringes were available. It was placed in the common metal cooler with the picnic food items sitting atop and among ice cubes.

When first bolting into my independence by leaving my mother's household, I carried my necessary insulin and syringes in a plastic sandwich-sized Baggie. This went on for years and years! Ziploc bags were not available as yet and became more secure with the storage of anything due to the plastic zipper. Great invention! In that 'traveling Baggie' was placed and stored at least two disposable syringes, insulin vials (2 of them because I was taking 2 separate types of insulin, NPH and Regular, that had to be mixed together), and rubbing alcohol-soaked cotton balls. Neatly put into my pocketbook, I was good to go. Road trips were easy with this 'private stash.' Although I oftentimes ignored the insulin having to be cold, refrigerated, I went on my way. They worked well for me. Today's inventive synthetic insulins seem to have to be refrigerated for their potency to remain. I did not go out of my way to refrigerate the NPH and Regular insulins that I used for approximately thirty years.

Airplane travel was easy, if not for being slightly embarrassed. My first air flight was to Florida for my honeymoon: warm beaches, poolside hotel room, Disney World, all good things. Before takeoff, however, I requested that the flight attendant "please place this parcel in the refrigerator. It's insulin." With forethought, I placed my 'baggie' supplies in a brown paper lunch bag with my name on it and the word "Insulin" written on the outside of the bag. No problem. Years later, and much to my delight, I purchased a specialized, hard plastic carrying case that would hold 2 bottles of insulin and 3 syringes. I still have and use it. Like an old friend, it's always there with a sense of security and familiarity.

Preceding flights continued in that manner until the Insulin Pump came into my life in 1996. Residing in California at this time period, California living introductions are forthcoming in Chapter 23.

My Diabetic Soul

When first purchasing the insulin pump device, it came packed in a clear, hard plastic briefcase-type carrying case with snap-up plastic hinges for opening and closing. At this writing, such a distinct item is no longer available. Therefore, I'll keep this case forever, another familiar friend. For your information, there are many different cases presently available for your convenience, at a price, and through research. In fact, due to my recent use of Apidra, I am in the market for an insulin case that will hold and fit these vials. They are a different shape and size from the previous insulin vials I have been accustomed to throughout my life to this point. I am on a mission to locate such a case.

Inside the hard plastic carrying case was not only the insulin pump but it's necessary accoutrements: batteries, battery covers that should, as I was told, be changed with every fourth battery change to ensure cleanliness; infusion sets; cartridges; adapter covers (that were suggested to be changed every tenth time that a cartridge is filled); needles to extract insulin from a vial for the cartridges; tape to secure the infusion set to the body; and the pumps' handy-dandy user's guide. Over the years, I upgraded certain items in my case to include IV3000 (a 2 ⅜" x 2 ¾" sized secure tape strips) as opposed to the adhesive tape I had used, pre-packaged tear-strip alcohol swabs, a cartridge "system" with needle attached, and a 'Link Assist' which is used specifically to aim and insert the infusion devices into my body at a straight, secure, angle. Inserting them by hand often caused the infusion to be crooked and bent. Not good. Bent needles not only disallow the insulin to be dispersed, but they hurt.

This case of necessities is then packed into my suitcase. However, for extra protection and peace of mind, I carry a small bag of one of each device in my pocketbook. One of two glucose meters is also in my pocketbook with its separate supplies. Once the refrigerated insulin pack is retrieved from a flight attendant, I am off to wherever I'm going, purposely placing the insulin pack in the refrigerator. I always ask for a refrigerator to be in my hotel room if that is my choice for overnight stays. As mentioned much earlier, during youthful family trips refrigerators were not always readily available. With that being the case, I would have to use the hotel sink to place my insulin, covered in ice. What a pain!

Gosh, I'm a lot of work!

Through the high security necessities due to September 11, 2001, my "stuff carrying" became a lot more complicated. At times, air flight travels were even embarrassing and humiliating. I'll explain:

On a flight from LAX (Los Angeles International Airport) to PVD (Providence International Airport, 2002), I was ready, organized, and anxious for many reasons. This was my first flight with my insulin pump and I was alone. Although I did not set off the beepers at the security check point, a physical scan redeemed the pump that was clipped to the front of my bra.

"What's that?" the young, female security attendant exclaimed as she walkie-talkie-radioed for "assistance with a female."

"It's an insulin pump," I replied.

"What's that?" she inquired further. Almost flattered at this inquiry, I explained "that this device delivers insulin into my body via computerized pump, automatically, as opposed to injecting it." Something like that.

"Show me," she said.

Well, I did, along with the rest of LAX, in front of the security camera. I pulled up my sweater and showed her. It was more like I flashed her and the rest of the world with my new and very comfortable royal blue colored bra. Memorable indeed! I was embarrassed, she was embarrassed, two other young, intense looking, female security officials were called forward. They lead me into a small adjoining room. In the meantime, all, I repeat – all – my traveling belongings were left at the initial check-point at the end of the conveyor.

"Take your clothes off," the tall, attractive yet scary blonde girl/woman commanded. I do not think she was more than thirty years old. I didn't take too much notice of the other one. I was scared.

"All of them?" I asked.

"Leave on your panties, bra, and socks" she coldly replied.

I didn't have to be told twice. Glad to be smelling clean and fresh, I stood there, becoming chilled, if only to state that "your concerns involve this computerized, medical device." Between the chill and my nervousness, I started shaking. I was not going to be probed!

"Let's see it," she demanded once again. The other young woman stood against the wall, viewing, witnessing.

Unclipping the pump from my bra, I handed it to her, explaining that I could shut it off and dislocate it from my body if necessary. With a white rubber-gloved hand, she held it, examined it, and gave it back. "Get dressed and go back to the security line," she commanded for the last time.

Once at the security gate, those two young women disappeared. I couldn't visually scan them anywhere, although I really didn't want to. The airplane waited for me. This had to take 20 minutes. Although nothing was said as I ran onto the plane, I was so-oo-o embarrassed from everybody looking at me, as if I was the culprit for their supposed impatient anxiety

I was never asked to provide the doctor's letter of which I secured with my medical belongings; I was never asked to provide proof of the medicines in my possession. I had also brought along extra prescriptions which are not unusual to be among my traveling paraphernalia. Gosh, I was just glad that that episode was over! Can you imagine? It never happened again. As the world became even more familiar with diabetes and its medical conglomeration of necessary collected and organized stuff, it was easier for me to fly. And I did. Phew!

"Who wants to go camping this weekend?"

A level of excitement was always raised in our household at such an announcement. Expectations were numerous: seeing long-time acquaintances, campfires with marshmallows, sleeping in a tent, using a sleeping bag, hiking, collecting pine cones and marbleized and shiny granite rocks and whatever else crossed our paths. Yes, camping is a close-knit family adventure.

With this in mind, let me pause and share another one of my genuine California traveling experiences with you, dear reader.

After a mandatory two-week reservation was made at a favorite campsite in Redlands, California, the planned packing begins. This is a lot of work! The inclusion of toiletries, linens, food items for 3 meals a day with snacks in between, weather watching, area event schedules, bicycle packing, and so much more (don't forget to bring logs and wooden matches for the fire pit!), is wearisome.

Well, one time I forgot my insulin. Good Lord! As I was using syringes at the time, the time was nearing for my 'bed time' injection. I couldn't find my insulin pack.

"Didn't you pack it in the cooler?" my husband nervously proclaimed.

"I thought I did. If it's not here, it's on the kitchen table" I nervously replied.

After looking through most of everything that I already looked through, 30 minutes went by. We concluded that it was not packed. The decision was made that we had to go to the nearest hospital, explain the situation, and get what I needed.

"Well," my honey said, "we could drive the two hours home to get it or find the closest hospital to get some. What do you have, like a prescription or something, to prove you're a diabetic?"

Hmm, it didn't take me long to think, but slower to answer "Nothing except my Medical ID necklace and my doctors' telephone number which is in my head along with my knowledge," I answered. It was the truth.

It was getting late. The campgrounds' information office would be closing soon. We hurriedly scrambled up the hill to that office, requesting directions to the nearest hospital.

Once there, the wait time in the emergency room was not long at all. It was more like waiting in a doctors' office library than the huge city hospital emergency rooms that I am used to. In fact, the whole hospital building was small. It housed no more than 34 patients at a time with a wholesome, clean country atmosphere. Its location, after all, was among farmland, in Small-Town, USA, where veterinarians would probably have been busier than human doctors.

Met by a young woman physician, her stern expression made me think I was going to receive a tongue-lashing or have to give up my first-born in order to get what I needed. Remember, I came there to request a weekend supply of a certain brand of insulin – with syringes. The "with syringes" part was the scariest.

My husband and I were brought in to a curtained cubicle typically reserved for sick emergency patients. "What is it you need?" she asked, with her eyebrows afloat.

"Insulin and syringes," I said. "I use [at that time] Regular with NPH, twice a day, a mixture of 30 units before breakfast and 8 units before bed. The disposable syringes I've been using for years," I went on, "are B-D ½ cc or 1cc."

She stared at me, listening intently, her dark eyes unmoving and fixed on my eyes. It was like she was reading the truth out of my soul by looking at me.

After more than a few questions, she made the long distance telephone call to my doctors' office. That was the longest part of this emergency room visit because it was a weekend. But, I passed! A nurse or assistant or whomever gave me a small brown paper bag, similar to a lunch bag, with the requested insulin and syringes inside. The doctor disappeared. However, as we exited the building, I could feel her glowing stare on me as I walked away. It felt as if there was just a subtle hint of mistrust in our encounter.

Since then, my reminder to not forget my insulin packet is to place some type of item – an empty insulin box, or an alcohol swab – purposely in my walkway. As soon as I see it, I know to grab the insulin for a trip.

Have you ever had insulin go bad on you? That's no fun either!

Another camping trip was highlighted through such an experience.

My husband and I were off to King's Canyon, an area in California where the Redwood Trees are too big to hug all the way around. Yes, I tried. They are marvelously gigantic! Sure, the tent, sleeping bags, pillows, change of clothes, toiletries, and cooler were all organized by yours truly. Yes, my insulin pack was packed as well. My insulin pump was less than half-full meaning I would and could re-fill the cartridge and change the usual attachments newly changed. The insulin pack, with a new battery, was stored in a Ziploc bag atop the ice with other fresh food items. I was ready. Not a problem in sight. We were both looking forward to this adventure. The smell alone of these beastly beauties was enticing and more inviting when I saw them reach through the sky to heaven. This forest gave all visitors a reason to look up and thank God for His Majesty! With a warm June breeze gently touching my skin as we surveyed the area for a camp site, I felt welcomed, at peace, this was meant to be.

The third day in this delicious Redwood Forest, my blood sugars began escalating. Here I go with the blessed signs again. Here I go with troubleshooting – again. Now my husband is involved asking me if the tubing is tangled; is it backed up with blood; when did I last change the battery; maybe the needle is bent; is there air in the line; on and on. We have become acclimated to expect the unexpected with or without the pump. Any other problems are unheeded.

Suffering through the weakness of high blood sugars and all that goes with that scenario, we got home, ready to call the doctor. "Wait," I told my husband. "Let me go through all the steps again, using a fresh bottle of insulin from the refrigerator." As this was my last vial, I would need to call the doctor for a fresh prescription anyway, but let me try to figure this out. I always prefer to figure my way out of a problem before having to ask for help.

Hours later, after I did the routine, my blood sugars leveled out. "That's it, hon," I proclaimed to my husband. "The insulin went bad. I'm never going camping again without a refrigerator. You can sleep on the ground with the trees and the stars. I'll be in a cabin or a trailer with a fridge. There will not be a second time. This was my sign."

Contacting my endocrinologist for a fresh prescription, I retold him my assumptions about the insulin. He agreed. It was as simple as that.

We did, in fact, resign to purchasing a 1.7 cubic foot refrigerator just for the gosh-darn insulin. Sure, it holds a few other things, making a camping experience more convenient. Nevertheless, keeping this synthetic insulin cool-to-cold is evidently of dire importance to me. Now when we go camping, it is with a pop-up trailer and my little fridge. Pieces of my mind and my peace of mind have been learned with expense!

While on a brief visit to see my friend, Suzette, I became violently ill. Vomiting with excruciatingly high blood sugars, my insulin just would not work. Not having brought my insulin and syringe kit along with me, I relied on my insulin pump. I felt confident enough with its use and purpose at that time and foregone any threat of an emergency. However, after repeatedly pumping up 30 or 50 units at a time every hour, this was ridiculous!

After a 1 ½ hour drive to get to her house, we went out to lunch and then dinner, arriving back at her home to watch a movie. Feeling a bit weird, I tested my blood; it was high – that is what the LCD (Liquid Crystal Display) screen read, "HI." Uh-oh. Thinking it must be due to the dinner (we both had had a chicken dinner with salad, mashed potatoes and broccoli, no dessert, at a nearby restaurant), I pumped up the jam. I was getting worse. Trying to nestle down for a night's sleep about 10:00pm, sleep wouldn't come. I pumped up more and my blood sugars rose. I was practically hysterical with fear!

At four o'clock the next morning I woke Suzette, telling her I had to leave, something was terribly wrong. She admitted that she wasn't able to fall asleep either and didn't feel well herself.

Even at that time in the morning, it took me two hours to get to where I needed to be - Torrance Memorial Hospital. During the drive I had to repeatedly pullover in the emergency lane to throw up.

Once in the hospital, I was diagnosed with food poisoning and ketoacidosis. Never in my life have I had either one of these conditions never mind having them at the same time! As defined on page 125, I was experiencing the presence and concentration of acetoacetic acid in my body. Not good. It doesn't even sound pretty! The word "acid" alone makes me think that my blood will start burning my body from the inside out resulting in a long and painful death. Yuck! I do not want to die that way!

The keto was due to my pump not working. Believe it or not, it failed on me. You see, before leaving my house, I was washing my face at the bathroom sink, nothing unusual, and a drop of water got on the pump. Knowing that this particular model was not waterproof, I quickly wiped the water spot away and thought nothing more about it. In the long run, that drop of water killed the pump.

The attending physician, Dr. Steven S., at Torrance Memorial was furious that this could happen and was even more infuriated when he telephoned the pump company and requested an immediate back-up pump be sent and that his request was refused. As told to me by him, he had to threaten them with a lawsuit. The pump arrived before the end of the day.

Oh my gosh, what a relief. Dr. S. delivered the pump to me himself, watched as I filled the cartridge and inserted the infusion set. He was more upset than I was but guarded me carefully. Gosh, I greatly appreciated his being there.

Before being released from the hospital four days later, I asked Dr. S. not to mention the ketoacidosis in my medical record. My record had been so unblemished until this time that I would have liked to keep it that way. I knew that that was an impossible request, but I tried.

Conclusively, two promises were made: neither Suzette nor I will ever eat at that restaurant again and I will never use that pump type again. That's the one I was talked into using in order for my endocrinologist at the time to be able to go to Hawaii. I went back to my trustworthy brand that supplies a back-up pump.

Another "Phew!"

Chapter 17
Welcome to the Machine!

"Welcome my son, welcome to the machine.
Where have you been? It's alright, we know where you've
been.
You've been in the pipeline, filling in time,
Provided with toys and Scouting for Boys.
You bought a guitar to punish your ma.
And you didn't like school, and you know you're nobody's
fool,
So welcome to the machine.
Welcome my son, welcome to the machine.
What did you dream? It's alright, we told you what to dream.
You dreamed of a big star, he played a mean guitar,
He always ate in the Steak Bar. He loved to drive in his
Jaguar.
So, welcome to the machine."
Pink Floyd - Album: <u>Wish You Were Here</u>

As satirical as these lyrics are, there is a dash of reality contained therein regarding diabetes.

Let me start with my familiarity with the machine known as a "glucomenter" (aka: "blood testing machine," blood machine," "blood kit," "meter," "blood meter"). I do not recall exactly when I began using a glucometer. Over the years, I have had many in my possession. Too many times such devices were freely given to me at one doctor's office or another. After many years of self-denial, these devices became more and more useful in my mature and thorough attentions self-care.

A. K. Buckroth

History of Blood Glucose Meters
By David Mendosa

"Starting at the very beginning, Ames developed and introduced in 1965 a product called Dextrostix®. These were paper strips to which you added a drop of blood, timed it for 1 minute and washed it off. They developed a blue color and you read that color by comparing it to a color chart. It gave you an approximation of the blood glucose level. People who did it on a regular basis got to read Dextrostix strips very well. But for most people because of limited usage you could know if it was very high or very low but in between it could be anything. Dextrostix were designed primarily for doctor's offices. Ames had been making urine strips and this was their first excursion into blood glucose strips.

"Then in 1970 realizing that the Dextrostix were difficult to use, one of the scientists developed a reflectance meter. That is a meter that could read reflected light."

I used the Dextrostix urine strips for a time, a short time, and was not fond of them. Too many times I peed on my fingers, having to hold one of these strips in mid-stream. You get the picture!

Along with this expensive, technical machinery, I carried specific and vital information of the utmost importance. Yikes! My record keeping would be of the *utmost* importance. This also meant I could stop using the *potty seat*!

At this writing, the FDA has approved the use of an insulin nasal spray. Having heard and/or read about this entrepreneurial invention, it has come to fruition. That's marvelous for those particular diabetics that absolutely do not, cannot, and will not inject themselves. Heck, I never had a choice. It was shoot up or die! However, a "nasal spray" device, full of insulin to spray up your nose is *not* appealing to me. The medication hits your brain real fast, then what? Consequences for everything!

My earlier mention of having to use an insulin pump for proper diabetic maintenance during a pregnancy has become old news at this writing. In fact, I purchased an insulin pump of my very own back in July, 1996. After feeling like I was going insane with out-of-control blood sugar readings and 4 – 5 injections *per day*, the decision was easy. Having read enough about them in many diabetic magazines available those days, I made telephone inquiries, did lots of internet research, spoke with doctors, etc., only to continue to be faithful to the name brand originally purchased – *Disetronic!*

The exertion of doing this research was tiring. However, I was sick. I wasn't right in my body or my mind. Essentially, nobody could or would help me. Nobody was available to understand or appreciate what I felt or what I was going through. My physician at the time was useless, again. Not only did he not know or care or understand or appreciate what I was feeling, he didn't know what an insulin pump was! My organs were suffering, I could feel it! My spirit was failing. My soul was crying. I HAD to do something! *I* had to do it, only me!

Back then, in 1996, the cost was $4,200 for two pumps and three days of training, three hours per day, in a conference room at a nearby medical facility. Because I "charged" it, I received a $200.00 discount. Whoopee! The next and updated version of a pump in 2006, through the same company, cost $6,200.00. No discount this time because my medical insurance carrier footed most of that bill.

As mentioned, two pumps were supplied. To my initial understanding, in order to maintain ongoing levels of care if one pump needed to be sent for calibration and/or malfunctioned, the other pump was available. And yes, the malfunctioning aspect has happened to me. Conveniently stored in a "medical closet" in my house, this second pump has been a life-saver!

For example, while vacationing cross-country, I experienced "pump perplexity," (aka: "failure").The attached machine constantly beeped and displayed "04" on its LCD screen. "04" means there is an "occlusion," a blockage. Well, having tapped it, changed the infusion set and body site, inserting new batteries, and whatever else I could do in my control, I finally called Disetronic technical support. Their telephone number is conveniently located on the back of each machine. I was told to change over to the second machine and send the malfunctioning one to the Minnesota office, the company's home-base. Well, I didn't have the other pump with me. This caused a telephone call to my husband back home that, in turn, sent me the necessary pump via Next Day FedEx. Phew! Since then I have never and will never travel without the extra pump.

I never did find out what went wrong with the original machine. I like to think and hope that is was re-calibrated and fixed up for a less fortunate diabetic person, anywhere in the world, who could not afford such a convenient device. I'll never know.

"We become bitter or better as a result of our experiences."
~ Eric Butterworth ~

The specific training for use of this particular insulin pump machine was more elaborate than what I received 16 years earlier for a successful pregnancy. With three buttons to control certain commands, and knowing the commands, the provisional booklet is a great reminder.

After speaking with a "General Medical" person about my initial request for an insulin pump, I was referred to Kaiser's one and only endocrinologist at the time. The fact of only one endocrinologist being available is stupefying to me! I will never understand that fact. But, that's what I was told and I had to see him to get a prescription for the machine. I need to mention that such a device was consistently and continuously advertised in the three diabetes magazines that were on my list of "have-to" reads (e.g. *Diabetes Health*, *Diabetes Countdown to a Cure*, *and Diabetes Interview*.) So, one day in June of 1996, I called the telephone number in the magazine article. That week – yes, that week – my husband and I met with a representative from the *Disetronic* Medical Systems, an insulin pump company. Her name was *Cindi*. Our meeting was scheduled at the convenience of my husband and me, in our home, in the evening, after work. Not only is Cindi a living, breathing, diabetic, but she has been on this brand of pump for eight years when we met! Eight years. That sounded like a long time, a 'too long time' to me.

Casual and introductory conversation told me she was married, had one daughter, lived 40 miles from us, had been diabetic for approximately 30 years at the time, and loved working with and for Disetronic.

She talked her talk and I put forth my credit card for the aforementioned $4, 200.00, with machine delivery within two days. As told to us by Cindi, that given price was discounted because I paid up front.

After a scheduled meeting with the aforementioned and particular Endocrinologist, the necessary prescription was promptly and personally turned in to the Kaiser pharmacy, specifically at the Kaiser Hospital in Harbor City, CA. After ten days, I received it and was directed to contact two nurses, "Susan" and "Suzanna." Susan, a juvenile diabetic herself, a nurse, and a pump user, was also an expert trainer. You see, as I was told, I was the first person under Kaiser's medical plan to use an insulin pump. Gosh, that made me feel special but quizzical at the same time. I could only hope that this experiment with myself would become an encouragement for others.

A pre-scheduled hour-a-day for three days, the three of us met in a conference room for my pump-use training. The training for use of this 3.5 ounce computerized machine began with adamant clarity to cleanliness (nothing unusual); use of alcohol swabbing of the area to prick or insert the needle (of which I still don't use alcohol swabs); filling of the cartridges (syringe part of the machine); the differences between "basal" rates and "blousing" (these words took me some time to ingest); the buttons to press separately or together in order for it to do what I wanted/needed the machine to do; and a gamut of many other commands. Mind boggling! Baffling!

Before I go any further, let me define "basal" and "bolus." A basal rate is "A continuous 24-hour delivery of insulin that matches background insulin need." In essence, via a computer command in the pump, the user has to program the basal rate. This is a per hour emission of insulin that is released into the body every three minutes. For instance, presently my basal rate profile amounts to 19.2 units of insulin per day. Every hour throughout a 24-hour period, the basal rate is programmed to emit 0.8 (eight tenths) of a unit of insulin every three minutes for a certain hour. This is also apt to change upon my command when necessary. When I have experienced instances of low or high blood sugars repeatedly throughout a number of days, the basal rate will be increased or decreased as to my discretion.

As to a "bolus," this is "A spurt of insulin delivered quickly to match carbohydrate intake or to bring a high blood glucose reading/level back to normal." With the distinguishing button on the particular pump I use, I press one to lead me to the option that reads "standard bolus." With that statement on the small LCD screen (2 inches x 1 inch), I have to press another button to get the spurt of insulin. For example, if my blood sugar is 220, I've been trained to know that I will need another two units of insulin to bring it down to 100. Therefore, I press one button to light up the LCD screen, another button to bring me to the standard bolus display, another button to accept that command, and still another button to put in the desired amount. As the measurement is in increments of tenths of one unit, that last button will need to be pressed ten times for one full unit.

Once the two units are calculated in a matter of 3 seconds, the insulin will be dispersed into my body. Depending on the amount of units, I can feel it. The larger the amount, the longer a burning sensation is felt. Usually, 6 units and more are felt.

(Accu-chek professional's pocket guide to infusion site management, © 2006.)

With all this quick training, I don't consider it to have been cost-effective. I did not understand or appreciate what I was being told at the time. That initiation was full of anxiety, nervousness, hypoglycemia as a result, and a forced hurried-ness to get the job done! I wondered if I should go back to becoming insane with plastic syringes every day or begin a new insanity with this machine attached to my body! I didn't. I learned through experience, taking my time, in my home element, to become comfortable with using this machine. I relented to being a cyborg! After all, this is a substitution as an artificial organ, my pancreas. And I am ever-so-acquainted with substitutions! There was promise with its use; the promise of a better and longer life, I don't know for how long, but I bought it.

The initial kit that was provided included small plastic bags with a piece of string through them. What the heck?! Well, these were to be used for showering – the pump goes into the bag wherein the bag is hung around my neck by the string and pulled tightly so as not to get the thing wet. Oh brother! Since then, the FDA has banned the pump from being near water. A great inconvenience in my opinion!

"So," you ask, "what do you do when you want to shower, bathe, swim, hot tub, or enjoy a water sport?"

Well, I shut it off first by pressing down two of the three buttons. Then I literally unhook it from my person. This means I have to untape the infusion set from wherever it is on my body, unhitch it from the plug-in site also on my body, and remove the whole thing, wrapping the tubing cord around the machine for safekeeping only to await the "re-plug." Keep in mind that I am only able to be without pump-infused insulin for an hour. I think you really have to see it to believe it and understand what I'm trying to tell you.

It's not much fun and water sports have become a disappointing, lost embellishment in my life. When in public, I no longer engage in delightful water activities because it is embarrassing and time consuming. Strategic thinking has to be involved along with the courtesy and kindliness of so many people that just don't understand. "Spontaneity" is not allowed.

For instance, one hot summer day, my daughter and I decided to treat ourselves with an ocean swim. She found a beautiful spot that would allow privacy before play. Well, so did many other folks have the same thing in mind! Sure, I ignored all but Heather as she watched what I had to do to disengage from this thing. It was – is –

tedious and time consuming. There was also my strategizing about keeping it safe, out of the sun and out of view of thieving eyes.

After a fair amount of water play, I had to return to the car and hitch myself back up. Over an hour had passed, and more time could have elapsed if I chose to ignore the needs of my body. Heather continued to boogie board and I became a happy onlooker.

Another similar experience occurred during a Hawaiian vacation. I *needed* to swim in the beloved Wiamea Bay. Having been there many years ago, I became briefly familiar with its beauty and longed to see it again, to feel it again, and to be a part of its beauty. Accompanied with my husband and tour-guide friend, Jonny P., we set out on a mission, a goal to visit Wiamea once again.

To make a long story short, I had to disconnect, store the pump properly, and hide it from curious eyes and fingers. You see, we were in a public area, having parked at least a quarter-of-a-mile away, and doing all this preparation in Jonny's tour van was unacceptable – to me. I wanted to get into that ocean as soon as possible, now, if not sooner.

Oh my gosh, what a feeling of freedom! I can hardly explain. The joy of being able to swim in the ocean, in Hawaii, in Waimea Bay, without encumbrances is pure joy! Pure joy! My husband and our friend were just plain happy for me, relieved. We accomplished this dream of mine together!

Unforgettable!

Until this manufacturer creates an insulin pump that is water-resistant, or better yet, water-proof, will I reinvest in another insulin pump. A "trade-in" is a good idea in my mind. However, trade-ins are not presently allocated or encouraged. Heck, I would think that the recycling capabilities of such an expensive machine would be feasible. Presently, that's just not the case.

Conjecture.

One thing I will never understand is the unique ability of Kaiser Permanente to oversee the Diabetes Insulin Pump therapy. Although at that time in 1996, the actual insulin pump became readily available albeit through a prescription *and* money if you had it. However, the other *many* necessities for its use and upkeep were not. Therefore, a middle-man (aka: other provider) was initiated. This company was known as "Apria Healthcare, Inc." The purchase of necessary supplies was not to be had at the Kaiser Pharmacy, only the specific type of insulin that I needed to use with it.

The constant necessities included infusion sets: a box of ten could last me 30 days. I say "could" because if I dropped one, it becomes un-sterile, thrown away, and replaced; or, if one becomes bent while in my body, it has to be removed and replaced. Yes, that happens often enough, spiking my blood sugar levels up like crazy because the insulin cannot get through the bent shaft and into my body! I find that such occasions depend on where the needle (infusion site) is located during my sleep. Hips and buttocks are bad places for me. You see, as a side-sleeper, I end up sleeping on the needle, awakening to an atrocious blood sugar (e.g., 326), feeling crappy, and having to change its location when I only did that the night before. On such occasions, I dig out an ol' friend, a shot, a syringe. Occasionally, the insulin pump infusion set tubing has become laced with blood and, of course, needs to be removed and replaced. Not pretty.

Due to the lack of body spaces/places in which to place these needles, I thought of putting one in my upper arm. After all, I used to use my arms for injections, so why not an infusion needle? Well, I took advantage of these arm areas for less than two years and had to stop. A burning pain running from the injection sites on upper arms through my armpits and into my nipples was a sure sign of nerve damage. I hit a nerve, probably numerous times, and had to stop. My upper arms are still healing at this writing, but I am considering using the areas again because *I'm running out of areas*. It's awful! I have dents all over my thighs, my buttocks, and my belly. Not pretty.

My personal medical supplies just for the diabetes upkeep take up space in a bedroom closet. This does not include regular band aids, or feminine supplies or aspirin. This bedroom closet shelf holds boxes and boxes of supplies that are used every other day. Because the infusion site needs to be changed every 48 hours to avoid infection, such items are necessary. And gosh, the paper trail is amazing. The packaging alone would raise the voice of an EPA (Environmental Protection Agency) agent!

Another necessity is the "transparent dressing," a type of adhesive tape sensitive to skin. It is used to hold the infusion set in place while it is in my body. Before these were introduced to me, I used white surgical or adhesive tape. Not only was those uncomfortable, but those types of tapes would become unstuck or unraveled.

Therefore, a box of 100 pieces of "IV3000 Adhesives" lasts 300 days. Keep in mind, once again, that the calculations *of the use of* these supplies are based on the theory that an insulin pump user changes the infusion set and site every 48 hours. That's not counting certain emergency situations. Confused? Well, that's okay. After a while, with practice, a person gets it all down to a tee! I did.

"Emergency situations" would include scenarios such as walking briskly past a door knob only to have the tubing catch on it and cause it to be literally ripped from your body. Nasty. Or, using the restroom and having it yanked out because of your pants. Or the clip, used to fasten the pump to a waist band, snaps free, causing the pump to plummet to the floor and yank itself out of your (my) body. Not good. There are other instances, but I'm sure you get the idea.

Another issue is *clothes*. A big part of my daily strategy is the wearing of clothes. As opposed to some of you that may be helter-skelter about this 'responsibility,' let's call it, I continually need to plan what to wear each day. Depending upon my body's infusion site, I dress for comfort with ease of accessibility. Imagine having to carry, clip, pocket, and wear your pancreas on the outside of your body. Everyday. My wearing of gowns or long formal dresses, especially skin tight has been difficult. The pump does not hide very well with sexy, revealing wardrobe pieces or formal wear.

As an example, my husband and I were invited to a semi-formal baptism with a following reception. Not wanting to have the pump bulging from the absolutely-adorable-dress I chose to wear, I stuck it into the pair of matching thigh high stockings. That was good – to start. Half way through the ceremony, it, the pump, started creeping down my leg with the stocking holding it close to my body. I started getting nervous; I started to sweat. "Oh my GOSH!" I'm thinking. "What do I do now?!" Keep in mind that we are in a Catholic Church with 144 other people.

Silently getting my husband's attention for assistance, he did a good job literally blocking me from sight in order for me to hand-walk this thing back up my leg and put it in another position – a comfortable position. Because I did not have its clip with me, I tucked the pump into the waistband of my underpants. Phew! That could have been mighty embarrassing! I laugh now.

Drama, drama, drama! I'm not and have never been a 'drama queen,' attracting attention to myself. Choosing to wear an insulin pump attracts its own attention!

Clipping the pump (plastic pump-clip purchased separately) to a brassiere front was a favorite place for me to wear it. That is, until a "spleen" pain episode halted this idea. This spleen pain story is explained further on. Therefore, the best spot is to clip it is on a waistband of whatever skirt or pant outfit I choose to wear. With this positioning, the weight of the pump eventually causes waist bands to wear out, threading thin. Underpants are replaced at least twice a year. Of course it can fit into a pocket, but not all clothes have pockets.

In essence, when I shop for clothes, which is rare, I need pants, dresses, skirts, etc. with pockets. Also tops with buttons or zippers are preferred for accessibility. It may sound easy, but it isn't when you're – I'm – looking for these specifics to include color choices, fabric choices, style choices, etc. So, I don't go shopping! It's become disappointing and fatiguing.

Sure, as with anything and everything, there are pros and cons. For instance, using a restroom takes just a little longer, if only due to having to unclip the pump, place it under my chin, gingerly remove my slacks or skirt, including the removal of stockings when appropriate, do my business, then put everything back in its proper and comfortable place.

In public restrooms, say during an event such as a concert or rodeo or ball game, I always feel rushed because the ladies restroom lines are always so long. Every girl and woman there is in need for a specific purpose. When I've rushed with the comfort of others in mind, I've had instances of accidentally pulling out the attached infusion, or had the infusion needle bend while in my body causing no delivery of insulin. Not good. This leads to a slow-but-sure-rise in my blood glucose level. I become uncomfortable with myself, uncomfortable with my surroundings and with anyone in my company. Easily within an hour of no insulin delivery, I become testy – moody – silent, tired to the point of wanting to sleep or take a nap or just rest. My brain doesn't register this at first. It's usually my husband that notices something just not right, asking "What's wrong?" I'll reply "I don't know. I have to test my blood."

With that simple question, I search out my glucometer from my pocket book, purse or sack, whichever may be with me at the time. Because of the weight of a glucometer, it always sinks to the bottom of any carrying bag making it an actual "search." Sure enough, my blood glucose level is a whopping 254 – or more – after starting the day at a beautiful and acceptable 108 or 118 or 154. With such a high reading (and yes, they've been worse, higher), I have to start the infusion troubleshooting process all over again. Sometimes we just go home.

Working up a nervous sweat, such occasions have meant exiting the arena or the fairgrounds or the mall or wherever. To exemplify the situation, the car has to be found to retrieve another infusion set along with its necessary condiments. Then, I once again have to take my time to locate a comfortable body spot, one without a dent, and insert it. Gosh, I'm thankful my husband is a patient man! I get so tired, so frustratingly tired. I want to be cured.

There have been instances when I look forward to a productive day with the infusion site comfortably, safely, and firmly in place.

My mind is on attaining a goal. However, the powers that be have had something else in mind, something to disturb my peace of mind. After a while, say a few active hours during a planned out busy day, it has became evident to me after too much moving around that the tubing that I so thoroughly tucked into my clothing became slackened causing an accident. Sure, it was tucked away well enough to conceal it, but my activity(ies) warranted a pause. When getting caught on such a thing as a door knob, as previously mentioned, the whole thing was yanked out of my body, causing a bloody mess. Or simply getting into my car, it has pinched and pulled.

More than a few awkward and rare instances have occurred when in haste, I quickly walked by a piece of furniture, or a car, or a simple pile of boxes, whatever, and pulled out the infusion set located in my hip or buttock. This was another one of those small but painful and bloody messes.

When either of these scenes have been portrayed in public, the drama in and of itself involves high anxiety: a search for a replacement infusion set (tubing), pressing on the area to make it stop bleeding, trying not to soil my clothes, and getting back to the dinner table, or wherever, calm and collected like nothing happened. Phew! When such instances have happened in the company of people other than my husband, the conversation turns into my being at fault with questions of "what, where, why, and how did you…"

It's not that the tubing is too long. I use the shortest one available at 24 inches. It's my haphazard attitude, or lack thereof, that gets me in any of these types of troubling situations. I am so used to wearing this thing that I take myself for granted thinking that everything is where it should be. Be forewarned if and when you are pondering the use of an insulin pump. Stuff happens for a reason.

The type of insulin used is peculiar to any insulin pump machine. Especially made with a buffer so as not to clog the tubing, the types of insulin I have used with my pumps have been Velosulin, Novolog, and Apidra.

More necessities include the plastic or glass cartridges to hold the insulin inside the machine's syringe case. 315 units is the maximum amount of insulin in any one cartridge which lasts me up to seven days. That's a good thing. While the cartridge may not need to be filled as often, the infusion sets *must be changed* every 48 hours. This action discourages infection. One cartridge of insulin will take me through 4 infusion sets, discounting emergencies.

Thus, I claim fame to being a cyborg. I walk around in life with a 3.5 ounce machine clipped to by belt, bra, waistband, or in a pant or skirt pocket that is both comfortable and big enough to hold it. A clear plastic tube no more than 24 inches in length dangles between the pump and my body site. This allows a life-giving and necessary human hormone to drip into my person every three minutes. If that's not a cyborg, I don't know what is!

Yes, it hurts at times. Placing the metal or plastic needle (aka: infusion set, catheter) inside my body is painful. Don't doubt it. Further pain is caused when bolusing insulin. Insulin burns. Taking the thing out to change it, as is necessary every 48 hours, causes distress as well. Oftentimes the needle site will bleed, swelling occurs, leading to painful scar tissue with bumps, and a bruise. Not too different from daily injections, if only because the results are the same.

Due to running out of spots to put the needle and being covered in lumps, bumps and dents known as "**lipoatrophy**," it is a loss of fat under the skin resulting in small dents and is caused by repeated injections of insulin in the same area. As with injections, the infusion sets are rotated in and around specific areas of a body and within any one site.

For example, specific body sites I have used are upper arms, waist area two inches away from my navel, lower tummy, upper thighs, back of thighs, and all of a buttock that I can reach without getting a side cramp. Within each of these areas, I imagine a circle. Throughout that imaginary circle are smaller circles wherein I place the infusion set – once. With six body areas to choose from, I scan the next area due to my rotation technique, safely placing the device.

Due to needles marks being left behind, it is easy for me to discern whether a certain spot is good to use or not. Forty-eight hours in any one area allows a previously used area to heal from former use.

Rubbing and messaging body site areas helps to break up the scar tissue in preparation for the next needle. It usually takes 6 – 12 days until a same site is rendered once again. For instance, with a "rotation method" in mind, place the first needle in your thigh somewhere. Then the next infusion three days later will be in the hip, buttock, lower belly or upper arm, staying in each area, one at a time, for three days. This is another part of the *strategizing* of this disease. Oftentimes the site hurts with sharp burning that I have to immediately remove the needle. That wastes a site. I get sad, depressed and often teary, having to choose another site. This is tiring, tedious; tiring is boring to me.

What cannot be helped must be endured."
~ Anonymous ~

Machines replacing for body parts, or parts of body parts, are nothing new. As a child, I wondered about the remarkable surgical insertion of pace makers. I don't recall how I first heard of such a thing. Nonetheless, it is another example. Another example might be a prosthesis. Although such devices do not supply a bodily fluid, they are necessary for progressive functioning of a body and its spirit.

Other examples could be: "Morphine drips" used to combat the pain of cancer victims; vocal cord mechanisms to allow certain people to speak when they otherwise could not; the placing of metal plates, screws, and/or pins in a body area to hold it together. I am not alone in survivorship. Yes, the "Ship called Survivor" could be a title for another novel!

So, man and machine have a history.

As recently portrayed through television commercials, versions of blood glucose monitors have gained attention and recognition. Thanks to such commercials, my secret is out. People that have seen me use such a monitor have immediately commented "Oh, you're diabetic." I am labeled as a "diabetic." I wonder what the stereotype is of a diabetic. A conversation always ensues with how the original commenter knows this person or that person – a relative, friend, spouse, child, cousin, etc. – has the disease and is either doing very well with a certain monitor or just the opposite, sometimes the *extreme* opposite.

These observations and their following conversations are out of control if only because the existence of this disease is out of control!

I have concluded that diabetes is boring. It's boring to me. I often divert the conversation to something concerning my profession or college or child or project. This disease has become boring; however the challenges are greatly alive. If I am one who has always lived with it and say that, I can imagine what non-diabetics think or feel. I think people are tired of hearing about it, funding for it and marathoning for it. This includes doctors.

Why not feel this way? This 21st Century, this magnificent number full of hopes from dreams and technology to come and imaginations with the encouragement of innovative creations becoming possible with expectations for a better everything for us all – has not, at least not yet. I am talking about a cure, a stop all, and an end all. I'm losing hope. I may have lost it all already. I have seen one sister suffer and die due to "diabetes complications." Another one suffers terminally because of this disease, and I deal with it every day, every tiring day.

Not to discount the myriad of other life-threatening diseases available, take your choice as to which one you would like to see cured first.

Alphabetically, as a world-wide society we have AIDS, Alzheimer's, Cancer, Chron's Disease, Colitis, Heart Disease, Huntington's Disease, Muscular Dystrophy, Parkinson's, Sickle Cell Anemia, Tay-Sachs, etc. Forgive me for not mentioning other diseases that you may have or be all too familiar with. Fill in the blanks. Poverty and greed may be added as well.

My question is: when will we see a cure for anything, for any of these? Not a treatment, not a pill, not a band-aid, but a cure! I continue to wait along with millions of others. Yes, millions, maybe trillions world-wide. Public anxiety continues to grow.

The following poem has been posted on the cork board in my office for many years. I don't recall where I found it and cut it from, but I laminated it and hung it above my work station and view it every day. It touched my heart and I want to share it with you:

Ode to an Insulin Pump
(from a grateful husband)

Sometimes, in the deep of the night
I encounter your tiny computer
lying between us,
its line tethered to your abdomen
like a spacewalker attached to the mothership.
The rustle of the down comforter
as you shift from one side to the other
cradling the little box
moving it, setting it down again,
a reflexive sound-asleep gesture to your little pal.
I've learned to appreciate
the insistent little beeps
when you disconnect,
leave your pump on the kitchen counter,
like a baby lamb's
plaintive bleats for it wandering mother
your little box, temporarily turned off
until blood sugars stabilize,
it nevertheless wants – need – to remind you,
"I'm here, ready...put me back in service."

I remember well the years B. P. (Before-the-Pump)
when I slept less than soundly,
always alert for the sounds of a low,

your wide-eyed stare,
the panicky times when you passed out, fell.
Your little pal
is now my little pal
affording me a good night's sleep,
much less worry.
Medical technology at its best
allowing you years of almost normal living,
lessening the onslaught of complications.
A blessing for both of us.
I can't even begin to imagine my life without you.
By Robert Lane, Oshkosh, Wisconsin.

"Corporate America" has become an issue with the curing of any disease. After all, and never doubt it, the bottom line is for them is making money. Remember, I'm a business major. My gains of knowledge made me acknowledge this fact. Stockholders want money. Government is a stockholder. *In my opinion*, pharmaceutical and medical companies are larger than the government. It is as if such companies, and others (e. g., insurance companies) dictate our Congress, our Senate, and on down the line. Politics aside.

In essence, what I want to say is that I seriously think we, as a world society, will never see a cure to anything because the costs of all medications for all symptoms, illnesses, diseases – whatever you want to call them – supports corporate spending. Skepticism has led me to become convinced that pharmaceutical companies in particular have abated cures.

For instance, excerpts from a particular article, title is below, was magnificently written by *Dara Mayers*. This has been fuel for my belief: there is a cure, there has been a cure for umpteen years now, but it is not being released due to the profitable monies being allied with the pharmaceutical industries. Along with the multitude of corporations, their tax dollars support the United States and its allies. Think about it. Corporations such as Bayer, Lilly (whom I grew up with, so to speak), Roche, Johnson and Johnson, etc., are household names. How did they get so big, so popular? Because you and I buy their products! I seriously would not doubt that every household medicine cabinet *in this world* has a product of one sort or another prescribed or purchased over-the-counter) by one or many of these huge, money-making manufacturing organizational corporations. Our dollars are thanks to them for chemically supplying us with chemically based, often poisonous and unnatural ingredients, which help to sustain our lives.

I am no different. The insulin I use is chemically manufactured. Therefore, my soap box isn't too big! And just like you, what choice do I have? Death is not a choice!

My personal suspicions were awakened many years earlier concerning the **billions of dollars** having been collected for *research of a cure of diabetes*. During my lifetime alone, including what I have personally collected for a "cure," doesn't measure up with my rationale of not getting what I need to cure this disease. I do not want or need another machine to sustain my life. I don't need to switch from machine to machine for the convenience of physicians who are often trained with and on one type of machine only. I have met many of them. I don't wish to wear another machine, meaning having to wear two infusion sets (needles) at the same time (e.g. the *GlucoWatch*) in order for *it* to detect another episode because it is supposed to be the 'biggest and best' innovation since time itself! I want a cure! My contempt has risen from scientific expertise. Mockery has assumed a public position of hindrance. How much more virtuous patience is necessitated for a cure?!

Too many time in my life have I found machines – devices - and then researched them, the numerous and varying types of medications (specifically insulin), dietary requirements, and everything else, by myself. It has been *very* rare, that a doctor/physician will inform me of something new and better toward my life's survival. I usually tell them! I have been diabetic for longer than most of my doctors have been alive, never mind their being doctors.

Quite a few physicians whom I have encountered throughout my life I have considered to be salesmen.

For instance, during one appointment or another, specifically for my diabetes care and prescriptions, the attending doctor has been excited, delighted and elated about sharing their latest knowledge about a new machine. Well, I don't take their gold star away from them. In fact, I am glad that they are learning. However, it comes down to the facts that so-and-so from this corporation or another is offering such-and-such if you agree to change your machine, or medication, or whatever. In my mind, the initial gold star is soon diminished.

You see, doctors/physicians have the ultimate trust of individuals at their fingertips. Theirs has always been a highly respected profession, a life saving profession. Rarely contradicted or challenged, doctors/physicians ultimately get paid for supposedly taking care of you and me. Life is important, right? And they get their perks, their incentives: a trip to Hawaii or Japan; free lunches; free prescriptions to hand out to their patients "to try." Be aware, dear reader.

Due to diabetics having the need to use numerous items to control their disease, to stay alive, to stay regulated and therefore, operate efficiently in this world, the individual and personal impact on the world economy is tremendously impacted and supported. Disease is a profitable market.

I feel there is a lack of integrity that is stupendously ignoble! It angers me greatly! Ms. Mayers beat me to the punch when writing the following article for the Diabetes Interview magazine years ago in 2003 that is emboldened below. However, my suspicions arose long before this article. I am glad that she had the wherewithal to be emboldened in this quest. Keep in mind this is one profitable disease among many, many others! I have had heated conversations with people of all ages concerning the belief that cures are just not going to happen, ever. I have not been alone with this opinion.

"Would You Cure a Profitable Disease?"

Here are excerpts from the article:

> *"In 1997, Lilly licensed INGAP, a protein discovered by Dr. Aaron Vinik of Eastern Virginia Medical School, which was deemed to have potential as a cure for both type 1 and type 2. INGAP causes the regeneration of beta cells in the pancreas, and many believe that it holds out promise as a truly innovative treatment for diabetes."*

> *"...In 1999, however, Lilly dropped INGAP from its portfolio. According to Vinik, it was not the science that the people at Lilly lost interest in."*

> *"They said, 'We love the science, but we don't think that it is a good business model," he said."*

The article goes on to read: *"Given the pressure for profit performance, it is unlikely that a pharmaceutical company would fund the basic science needed to find a cure. It just isn't a good investment decision."*
(www.DiabetesinControl.com.)

As mentioned early about machines, the competition and marketing of health *aids* has grown tremendously over the years. The cost of all devices costs the consumer big bucks. How is this money allocated, specifically, when multiplied by the 24 million + diabetics using all this stuff? Hmm.

Diseases – diabetes – is a billion-dollar-a-year money maker, don't doubt it! Rationally, why would any researcher or research company even be allowed to boast of a cure?! Why would healthcare teams and systems along with world-wide pharmaceutical agencies want to cure it? They don't. I don't believe they do. Instead, more and more devices are invented to "control" diabetes, to allow the diabetic just a little piece of mind in thinking that "I'll be all right. I'll live long enough to attend my grandchild's wedding." Nope. These devices are a scam. They are "band aids." I am thoroughly convinced.

Realistically, a cure to any of our world's diseases would put an end to the cash flow! It could very likely lead specialized doctors, physicians, researchers, etc. into other careers, new jobs.

Change brings chaos and chaos brings change.

My advice? Take care of yourself. Use whatever machine is comfortable. Use the so-called "band aids." Listen to your health care providers. You're in control. Research for yourself. Be pro-active. Remain on top of the knowledge information freeway. Be as happy as possible. Learn, learn and learn some more. Be active, not just physically, but mentally and spiritually as well! We're all this together, with or without a disease. Let's help each other!

Over the course of many, many years, I had heard about or read something or other about "*NIH*" or "*NIDDK*" and others. What are these? They are corporations, organizations, if you will. "*NIH*" stands for "National Institutes of Health" and "NIDDK" for "National Institute of Diabetes and Digestive and Kidney Diseases." This last one sounds impressive yet intimidating. Visually, what comes to mind when I hear these abbreviations are extremely tall, shiny glass skyscrapers consisting of about 52 floors, each full of office equipment and people. What do they do? Who knows? What does it cost? A lot. Who pays for all this, inside and out? We do, the taxpayers, the working stiffs. You and I hear *of* them but not too much *about* them. There is a difference.

Both organizations boast of research, but what does that mean? The word 'research' is so loosely and widely used. My best imagination calls forth a vision of men, mostly, dressed in laboratory coats over dark pants with dark leather shoes. Most of these researchers in my imagination are pictured as being older, say 55 years old, have their hair neatly trimmed off the collar, clean shaven, tidy, and are too serious. Many of them wear glasses, some with hanging chains for easy slip on and off, and a pocket protector for pens in a breast pocket. Do I watch too much TV? Maybe. My imagination continues to place each of them in front of a microscope atop a shiny, cold, metal counter that has metal drawers and cupboards below for storage. For every 3 – 5 researchers/scientists, there is a female assistant. And you can take it from here…

As I have never seen a research facility but heard about them over and over again, I can only conjure up this visualization. Imagination at play.

As the NIH and NIDDK seems to be a large 'umbrella,' this may allow each to form smaller working groups (e.g., one for Type I Diabetics, one for Type II Diabetics, another for Beta Cell functioning or mis-functioning, Islet Cells, Stem Cells, etc.) *DAISY* is one. An acronym for "Diabetes Autoimmunity Study in the Young." The *JDRF* (Juvenile Diabetes Research Foundation) and the CWDF (Children with Diabetes Foundation) are others.

With the above mentioned research teams underway, the processes remain baffling and endless. Continually funded through private donations (e.g. money-raising marathons, 3k, 5k, 10k walks; government grants and allotments, etc.) they survive as non-profit organizations are a free from paying taxes. But that's not the point here. Will it ever stop? Research, research everywhere, not a cure to be found. I'm still waiting.

Early one spring evening of 2009 my cousin, Randy, telephoned me. As unusual as this was in and of itself, he was greatly excited. He needed to me of an available cure "for everything!" Oh my GOSH! Sure, he got my uninterrupted attention.

"A guy I work with," he began, his wife has cancer. I don't know where her cancer is or what type it is. But he brought her to a place called "Medra" and she's undergoing treatments and is almost cured."

"Things that make you go Hmm," I thought.

"Check it out" he demanded. "The place is called Medra. They have a 1-800 number. My friend told me to tell *you* about it. It could be worth your while. It's been advertised on the radio." Well, okay then! What more substantiation did I need? None!

Immediately, I rushed to my home-office computer, sat down, took a breath thinking "Could this be true?! Could this be true?!" Typing in the word "M-E-D-R-A," the Google search came up with a full website. Calling the 1-800 number shown on the website, I left a message. While doing all of this, I kept asking myself why hadn't I heard of this? Well, in answer to my own question, I do not listen to news-talk-radio. My bad.

To make a long story short, "Medra" is a medical facility that delivers "the future promise of Fetal Stem Cell Therapy today. Founded and lead by Dr. William Rader,...Medra has offices and laboratories in California U. S. A, Georgia (The Former Soviet Republic), and Germany....The treatment consists of a transplantation of Human Fetal Ste Cells,...is performed on an out-patient basis.,...taking one hour,...costing $30,000.00,...within a private treatment center in the Caribbean." (**http://www.medra.com**.)

Golly gee, I would like to go to the Caribbean. However, not for $30K! I let it go. Since Randy's telephone call, I have still never heard of such a thing or a place or the doctor. Gosh, that little light of mine was almost sent bursting through the skies! Hope seems to find me when I least expect it.

Chapter 18
Afflicted

While certain of the aforementioned television advertisements for blood monitors have proclaimed them to have a "painless" usage, that's not true. Rationally, how can it be? The user has to draw his or her blood in order to test properly. It's impossible to make yourself bleed without pain! In my experience, they are painless if only because a long-time user has lost feeling in his or her testing sites (e.g., fingertips and/or the inside of arms, even earlobes!). Oftentimes this is a cause of neuropathy, a deadening of the nerves, especially in outer extremities, due to poor circulation. Nerves become damaged. Period.

> *"**Neuropathy** is a medical term referring to disorders of the nerves of the peripheral nervous system (specifically excluding encephalopathy and myelopathy, which pertain to the central nervous system. It is usually considered equivalent to peripheral neuropathy, which is defined as deranged function and structure of peripheral motor, sensory, and autonomic neurons, involving either the entire neuron or selected levels. According to some sources, a disorder of the cranial nerves can be considered a neuropathy.*
>
> *Neuropathy should not be confused with neuropathology, which deals with the pathology (i.e. the study of disease and disease processes) of nervous tissue."*

Having become effected and diagnosed with "peripheral neuropathy" toward middle age, I had to fight to get monetary assistance with the Social Security Administration. I could no longer work. I was in too much pain. It hurt to accomplish minor tasks and responsibilities such as typing, lifting, reaching, pushing, pulling, etc. After four years of applications, denials, court appointed doctors, nerve conduction studies, weeks of physical therapy, letters from family and friends concerning my health decline and, finally, legal representation, I was awarded. That process was brutal. The career was brutal and gladly coming to an end. I just couldn't do it anymore.

The monthly Social Security allotment alone would not afford me to live in a trailer, never mind the beautiful ranch house I presently occupy with my husband. If it wasn't for him and his 'breadwinning' capabilities, I would be homeless! As I tell him as well as family and friends, I am expensive if only due to medical costs.

It wasn't easy! Perseverance took over my soul with a dire need to live, subsist, with money. I wouldn't survive being homeless. Having already learned respect of money, or lack thereof, after 'being on welfare' those many years ago, I knew I would never be rich, or 'well-off.' After all, I am a working class girl, always have been, and was raised that way. Limitations and sacrifices of many things in this life was not, is not, isolated or surprising.

Continuing with this topic, the following letters, addressed to *my* representative at a Social Security office, is a request for an appeal after being denied assistance for the third time. This was a time in my life when I truly learned what a bureaucracy was – and was not. If anything, my definition of a bureaucracy is room, although could be a building, full of people shuffling one paper to another, causing an inefficient waste of time and tax payers' money. It's not a good thing.

In these letters, names and numbers have been deleted for apparent reasons.

February 21, 2001
Ms. Linda _____

Regional Commissioner
Social Security Administration
336 North Gaffey
Suite 101
San Pedro, CA 90731

RE: Claim Number: ___-__-___HA
        SSA Pub. No. __-_____

Dear Ms. _____:

In recognition of your letter dated February 14, 2001, concerning ineligibility for benefits, consider this letter as a written *"Request for Reconsideration", as required, of the above case.*

I disagree with this decision via the "Notice of Disapproved Claims" due to the facts in my medical file. The acclaimed and chronic "Low Back & Waste Pain" constricts me from walking, standing, sitting, and sleeping. Dr. Sushila A._____, M. D. and Primary Care Physician through my medical insurance policy, has been repeatedly and consistently told of my painful predicament over a course of a few years. These facts should clearly be noted in my medical file in her possession.

Also, Dr. John T.____, Endocrinologist, has communicated certain factual findings of this pain and his concerns for my diabetic status.

As listed in my original application form in December, 2000, my bodily discomfort is not limited to the lower back and waist areas. Others include "Frozen Right Shoulder" causing constant pain and immobility of right arm; constant discomfort to both hands and wrists due to "Carpal Tunnel Syndrome" and "Diabetic neuropathy". These facts are in my many various and vast medical filings through a team of approximately seven (7) physicians.

Pain cannot always be seen. But pain certainly can only be felt! As an attractive middle-aged woman, people - all people - have denied me such *the possibility* of constant pain. Society does not admit that beauty and pain are acquainted. Faced with diabetes for fifty years, people – physicians included – have been repeatedly shocked that I possess all my faculties and body parts! However, they do not see the constant pain and discomfort that I have trained to operate and function as a human being on a daily basis. I hurt. It hurts me to acknowledge that physical beauty is a hindrance to being disabled.

Therefore, I anticipate hearing from you and/or a staff member to sign the necessary SSA-561-U2 form. In the meantime, if for any reason pertaining to this appeal you may want to contact me, please do so during business hours at **(310)___-____**.

Thank you in advance for you kind attentions to this matter.

A. K. Buckroth

bc: Mrs. S. D._____
cc: Carolyn W. _____

August 19, 2001
Linda_____, Regional Commissioner
Social Security Administration
Suite 101
336 North Gaffey Street
San Pedro, CA 90731

RE: Claim Number ___-__-____ HA

This is a request for a listing of other disability programs in the State of California, both government and private.

This letter is due to consistent unanswered telephone calls made by me to **310.___-_____** and **1.800.___-_____** for the aforementioned information.

In a letter to me from your office with your name dated April 26, 2001, page 2 of 4, expresses "that there are many types of disability programs, both government and private, which use different rules."

Therefore, I would like your assistance in locating these organizations. I need financial assistance and am not employable due to constant pain and being under the care of many physicians.

Sincerely,

A. K. Buckroth

cc: Mrs. D_____
         American Diabetes Association
         Alexandria , VA

         International Diabetic Athletes Association
         Phoenix, AZ
         American Association of Diabetes Educators
         Chicago, IL

         Joslin Diabetes Center
         Boston, MA

         International Diabetes Center
         Minneapolis, MN

         American Dietetic Association
         Chicago, IL

         American Heart Association
         Dallas, TX

         Nat'l Foundation for Depressive Illness
         New York, NY

         Nat'l Institute of Diabetes And Digestive and Kidney Diseases
         Bethesda, MD

         Juvenile Diabetes Foundation Int'l
         New York, NY

At the same time, I thought it appropriate to contact the American Disability Association. I was looking for help, some type of assistance. Therefore, this particular letter I diligently composed for a purpose.

September 10, 2001

REQUEST FOR ASSISTANCE
BRIEF SYNOPSIS OF FACTS

American Disability Association
Member Services
2201 Sixth Avenue South
Birmingham, Alabama 35233

To Whom It May Concern:

In my personal efforts to gain disability assistance, I have had no other choice than to contact your organization directly. The attached letter has gone unheeded and further adds to my anxiety. I am hoping that the American Disability Association can refer my energies to the proper authorities.

You see, I have been a diabetic since 1959. Over the past decade, persistent/chronic back pain, pain in both shoulders, arms, and wrists have prevented me from performing normal and menial daily tasks. Much of this is due to the complications of diabetes – peripheral neuropathy, carpal tunnel syndrome, with subcutaneous ligament tears.

Having filed for Social Security Disability benefits earlier this year, it was "determined that my condition is not severe enough to keep me from working." However, that organization has not encouraged me to seek other estuaries of information.

Therefore, I ask for your assistance and/or references to the proper agency(ies) in order for me to gain some type of monetary assistance. My suffering is prolonged without a financial income. As displayed, the schedule of appointments for 2001, this far, would interfere with any career manifestations! Time consuming as they are, these appointments do not reflect travel time nor its expenses. It gets to be pretty scary when a person has no income!

If necessary to gain your attentions, I will be more than glad to assist in the efforts of gathering medical information. Much of it is already organized in my personal records.

Sincerely,

A. K. Buckroth
Street Address
City, State, Zip Code
310. ___-____

Attachments

2001 Personal & Mandatory Physician Appointment Schedule (see following page).

Attachment

2001 Personal & Mandatory Physician Appointment Schedule

Jan 3	Physical Therapy	Mar 29	Surgery	Jun 22	Dr. Peters	Aug 20	Dr. Arnette
Jan 29	Dr. Lee	Apr 10	MRI	Jul 3	Dr. Millman	Aug 22	Dr. Arnette
Jan 31	Physical Therapy	Apr 12	Dr. Kwon	Jul 5	Dr. Pachman	Aug 22	Dr. Co
Feb 13	Dr. Singh	Apr 13	Dr. Herring	Jul 5	Dr. Harwood	Aug 27	Dr. Arnette
Feb 14	Physical Therapy	Apr 19	Dr. Tuey	Jul 11	Physical Therapy	Aug 29	Dr. Arnette
Feb 16	Dr. Guba	Apr 20	Dr. Herring	Jul 13	Physical Therapy	Sept 4	Dr. Arnette
Feb 19	Ultrasound	Apr 23	Dr. Herring	Jul 19	Physical Therapy	Sept 5	Dr. Arnette
Feb 21	Physical Therapy	May 11	Dr. Pachman	Jul 23	Dr. Herring	Sept 6	Dr. Tsao
Mar 1	Dr. Kwon	May 14	Dr. Tsao	Jul 24	Dr. Arnette	Sept 7	Dr. Arnette
Mar 1	Dr. Singh	May 16	Mammogram	Jul 27	Dr. Kissell	Sept 10	Dr. Arnette
Mar 12	Dr. Tsao	Jun 4	Dr. Herring	Aug 1	Dr. Co	Sept 11	Dr. Kim
Mar 16	Dr. Herring	Jun 7	Dr. Pachman	Aug 13	Dr. Arnette	Sept 12	Dr. Arnette
Mar 22	Dr. Agrawal	Jun 7	Dr. Tsao	Aug 15	Dr. Arnette		
Mar 27	Dr. Kwon	Jun 11	Dr. Herring	Aug 20	Dr. Kissel		

Chapter 19
"Doctor, doctor, give me the news."

Getting back to my theory that doctors are bored with diabetes has been proven to me, personally, time and time again. And why not? My answer to that is because there are just too many diabetics, each one different as personalities and lifestyles are different.

For instance, with the onset of insulin pump use, in the thirteen years of using this device I have not, as yet, found a doctor that is familiar with it, especially the one I use. Literally, I have shown, displayed, and literally taught them about its uses. If I thought looking for a diabetologist to sharpen my tools toward better health was difficult, looking for an endocrinologist familiar with insulin pumps is another challenge!

Diabetic patients are passed on to other professionals, care givers and/or "diabetes team workers" as they are referred to. Doctors are needed to prescribe what is needed for a patient, according to the patient symptoms and/or distress. I am a patient. I have been a patient all my life. My medications, tools for survival (e.g., diet, or lack thereof, insulin dosages, exercise routine(s), and stress level(s)) have been researched and monitored *by me*. When I have informed one doctor or another of my routine, certain symptoms of concern, or other factors pertaining to *my diabetes*, I get brushed off. No comment is made. I have been ignored. Such results are ignorantly alarming and lead me to search for a more knowledgeable doctor.

For instance, another "diabetes sickness" known as the "dawn phenomenon" entered my life during my mid-to-late thirties. Terribly confused as to why my before bed blood sugar readings were normal only for me to awaken with a high reading, a *very* high reading, I posed this circumstance to my doctor at the time. Alarmed, I did not understand. Once again, I blamed myself for having don – or not done – something to initiate the highs. This happened over and over and over again. Once I explained this to my endocrinologist, he remarked "Oh, you're experiencing the Dawn Phenomenon."

"I don't know what that is," I cried.

He then replied "I want you to go to such-and-such a class. You'll learn about it there."

Well, I did not want to go to a class. Why couldn't he just explain it to me? So I looked it up myself. It does not only happen to diabetics. Such a thing occurs with many, but not all, people. It has to do with hormones being released while we are asleep. How simple. Why couldn't the doctor just tell me that! There are ways to avoid it as well: lower my carbohydrate intake during my evening meal and no eating (for me) after 7:00pm.

All in all, I found the doctors' attitude to be quite ignoble, lacking care. I felt that he did not want to be bothered. Due to medical insurance affordability issues and the aforementioned proper treatment, the opportunity to leave that medical program arose and we opted for another. With some research, again, and a referral, an endocrinologist was located near home. "Near home" is always a good thing.

It was during this time that the term "Ace Inhibitor" was introduced to me. Without a lengthy explanation, this particular doctor prescribed such a drug.

"What's an Ace Inhibitor?" I asked.

"It will keep proteins out of your urine," he replied.

"Oh, okay," I thought. For one, I was not made aware that I had proteins, plural, in my urine. For two, I did not know the dangers of such a factor. I did not know too much on this subject and I certainly was not going to ask him! I already felt like I was putting him out of his way. So, my pro-active research taught me.

Briefly, such a pill slows my blood pressure which, in turn, lowers the pressure in the kidneys. It is supposed to slow the progression of kidney disease, a frightening high risk factor with diabetics. I don't want kidney disease. I'll take the pills, every day, for the rest of my life. This began in 1997.

Back to the topic of doctors being bored with diabetes, this is a most recent, personal example. I experienced a sharp and consistent pain under my left rib-cage. Thinking I over exerted myself with leaf raking one Sunday in May, 2007, perhaps pulling or twisting a muscle or tendon, my typical home remedies – the use of ice packs and then heat via a hot tub and heating pad - I immediately contacted our family chiropractor, Dr. James S. As usual, even at the late hour it was, Dr. S. helped to mildly relieve this initial throbbing pain.

Having procrastinated long enough to visit my regular endocrinologist, Dr. Conrad T., I made an emergency appointment. Dr. T. and I have been acquainted through my healthcare system since re-locating to this area some years ago. This 'emergency appointment' on November 1, 2007, left me in the waiting room for three hours. To make a long story short, he talked me into his giving me a shot of a numbing solution in order to see if this pain is muscular or something more serious – an organ. Due to my own research, I've been calling it "my spleen pain" because the pain is precisely in that area. In my frightened state of anxiety, I also suspected that something is wrong with my pancreas.

Numbed, I went home. An hour and twenty minutes later, the pain was there, as bad as it ever was. Calling Dr. T.'s office once again, I had an appointment for November 8th. *My* main purpose to see him, again, was to request orders for a MRI as well as get a pain medication. I would really like to find out what the *cause* of this pain is! Well, that appointment was deflated if only due to having waited an hour. Angry, and in pain, I left. I didn't want to sit there for another 2 hours!

In the interim, I had already made a big decision to become involved with the world-renowned University of California, Davis, Medical Facility (UC Davis). Hoping to make an appointment with the acclaimed Endocrinologist and Professor, Dr. Thomas A. whom I had read about, that did not happen. You see, my rationale for making this BIG decision had big hopes. I filled my brain full of bright and shiny ideas of diabetic revelations! I could teach them a thing or two, I was sure, and vice versa!

Instead, on November 9, 2007, my husband and I met with Dr. Allen T., Resident Intern at UC Davis. Realizing that UC Davis is an academic hospital, getting to the top dog is strongly un-encouraged. Disappointing at best.

Besides wanting to become set-up and familiar with such an important institution, I lowered my expectations, thinking that somewhere along the line during this visit the esteemed Dr. A. would magically appear to see someone as important as I. That was a laugh.

Meeting Dr. Allen T. was delightful enough. My first impressions were that he is young, ambitious, a listener, and a newbie. For his specific review, I prepared a one-page biography of my health background. That's not unusual for me. I try to be open-minded and objective when presenting myself, especially in this case – the need and want of expert medical attention. I went on to explain the 'spleen pain' to Dr. Allen T. During this initial examination, he invited Dr. Kevin K. into the room. Although poked and rubbed once again, nothing was found.

Oh, woe-is-me!

A requested MRI was denied, again, along with a denied request for an X-ray. Although I believe an X-ray would be useless because of the soft tissue involved, I also believed with hope that anything would help. Happily, a "CT Abdomen with contrast" was arranged and performed on November 21st. It showed nothing pertaining to *this* specific pain. How can that be?! However, it did show *other things*. These "other things" were not addressed, but totally ignored such as an ovarian cyst and a displaced disk. It appalls me that nothing, nothing, nothing was said to address these issues. I don't get it! This consistent ignorance has always lead me to do my own research for cause and effect. Without the internet as a research unit, I would have to live in a library or form one of my own! Information is knowledge! But, one thing at a time. I need to focus on this "spleen pain."

After a year and a half, the pain persisted. As described to anyone who would listen to me, medical personnel or otherwise, it felt like a knot, a golf ball, under my front left rib cage with numbing of the whole left rib area. Like a large marble is stuck. The pain is stronger when I eat, no matter what I eat and the pain also strengthens when my blood sugars are too high (high being 185) or too low (low being 75). Any ideas? In the meantime, I'll be back at physical therapy to see if this cannot be "stretched out."

So far I have seen six (yes, eight) doctors/physicians concerning this issue at the UC Davis facility! Along with Drs. Allen T. and Kevin K., there were Drs. Allen T. with R.; then Allen T. with O'.; then Allen T. with 'can't remember his name!'

A painful emergency rib situation brought me to and through an 'urgent care' appointment at the University of California Davis (aka: UC Davis) in Sacramento, California. I had an attack of that "spleen pain" again! On a scale of 1 – 10 with 10 being the worst, this pain was a 10, sharp and distinct without cause. It felt like the thin sharpness of an ice pick was being pushed in that spot. The wait wasn't as long as I expected, wherein my husband and I were met by Dr. G. Being under the impression that such a predominant "research facility" would be beneficial in more ways than one, I chose, with very high hopes, to check it out. After all, I compared it to my beloved University of Massachusetts (aka: UMASS).

"What brings you here today? Something about ongoing abdominal pain?"

"Yes," I replied, and continued with the truth of my story beginning on May 9, 2007.

"Any vomiting," she asked.

"No, but I do experience occasional nausea. And dizziness."

"When do you get dizzy?"

I replied "Most usually when getting out of the shower or hot tub."

"Oh, okay," she said. "That is typical [blah blah blah] blood pressure." I remembered agreeing.

"Blood in your urine or feces?"

"No. And I notice the pain worsens during and after eating. No matter what I eat. It is especially worse when my blood sugars are too high (e.g., 185) or too low (70)."

She asked me to repeat what I just said in which my husband agreed and backed me up.

After a mid-section, front and back examination, she took a seat, looked at us, and said "I think it could be a blocked intestine. (Key words: "I think it could be.") "That CT scan [dated many months ago, mind you] was inconclusive due to fecal matter. Please wait here. I'm going to discuss this with Dr. H., my attending physician tonight. Okay?"

"Okay, fine," I said. "That'll make a total of eight doctors that have seen me, since November, about this pain. Not only Dr. Allen T., but also his 'attending physicians.' There has been Dr. Conrad T. before coming here, than Drs. Allen T. with Kevin K., then R., (cannot remember his first name), and now you [Drs. G. and H.]. I'd like to find out the cause of this pain, not just treat the symptoms."

"Yes, I know," she replied. "You've seen a lot of us."

"Heck," my husband proclaimed! "This could be an episode on 'House' (a television show at the time). That comment brought a chuckle to us all. "Also," he continued "she drinks fennel tea that alleviates some of the pain."

"Well, continue drinking it," remarked Dr. G.

With that, she excused herself saying she would discuss the symptoms and return with her attending physician, Dr. H.

Not 5 minutes later, Dr. G. was accompanied with Dr. H.

All in all, it was decided, and concurred, that I have something known as "*gastroporesis.*" Therein a prescription was written up for 5 mg of '*Reglan*' to be taken 30 minutes before each meal.

I didn't like hearing that. Remember, I'm not a pill taker. Immediately concerned, I mentioned already taking *Benazapryl* and (useless) *Lipitor.* My husband piped up with the possibility of 'side-effects' question.

"Also" began Dr. H., "I've put down for you to have a Barium CT

Scan. This will show what's going on in that specific area."

"Halleluiah!" I wanted to scream! "Finally! A doctor that believes me, that wants to find out specifically what this pain is!

Dr. H. mentioned the possibility of *gastroporesis*. That is *not* what I wanted to hear! More internet research brought me to the following definition and cause:

"Gastroparesis, also called delayed gastric emptying, is a disorder in which the stomach takes too long to empty its contents. Normally, the stomach contracts to move food down into the small intestine for digestion. The vagus nerve controls the movement of food from the stomach through the digestive tract. Gastroparesis occurs when the vagus nerve is damaged and the muscles of the stomach and intestines do not work normally. Food then moves slowly or stops moving through the digestive tract."

What causes gastroparesis?

"The most common cause of gastroparesis is diabetes. People with diabetes have high blood glucose, also called blood sugar, which in turn causes chemical changes in nerves and damages the blood vessels that carry oxygen and nutrients to the nerves. Over time, high blood glucose can damage the vagus nerve."
(Wikipedia, the [Internet] free encyclopedia.)

Getting ahead of myself at this juncture of the story, I must share with you that, so far, I have had three prescriptions for this pain: "Levsin, 0.125 mg to be placed under the tongue every six hours as needed [for pain];" "Metoclopramide," 5 mg taken orally 3 times a day (30 minutes before meals); and "Gabapentin," 300 mg, one capsule taken at bedtime. What the heck are these?!

"Levsin is used to treat a variety of stomach/intestinal problems."

"Metoclopramide is primarily used to treat nausea and vomiting, and to facilitate gastric emptying with patients with gastroporesis."

"Gabapentin was originally developed for the treatment of epilepsy, and currently is widely used to relieve pain, especially neuropathic pain."

As mentioned much earlier, I am not a 'pharmaceutically engineered' pill taker so repeated dosages was really quite difficult for me to adhere to. Levsin had an immediate effect of pain relief that lasted *maybe* 30 minutes. The Meto… stuff I was able to follow through for two days. I never remembered to take it, it was a bother, I didn't want it. My bad. Those two days when I did swallow it before meals, I was given temporary pain relief. *Temporary* meaning the pain faded only to return ever stronger. And the last, the Gabapentin, caused me diarrhea for eight days. No thank you! Eight days is a long time!

And I'm not done with this part of my story.

The "Barium CT Scan" was a farce. It never happened. Allow me to explain.

Reporting to the UC Davis Medical Center via an appointment, my husband and I arrived early. We both had hopes of walking to a nearby restaurant for a quick breakfast. A breakfast burrito was on my mind. However, the attendant started explaining that he "will fix me some eggs and toast. As soon as I'm done eating, the test will begin." I was shocked! Here I was expecting a dye injection or the necessity of drinking the nasty, chaulky tasting barium when that was not the case at all. Unbeknownst to me, the test ended up being a "gamma test."

You see, while the food is ingested and on its way through the esophagus to the upper intestine to the stomach, etcetera, I had to stand in front of a large metal scan that taped all this action. Painless and interesting, it bothers me to know that I was not told that that was going to happen. Good thing I didn't eat before we left the house! This instance was another 'divine intervention.' Not only did my husband take the morning off from work, because there were three parts to this scan. Each scan was approximately 45 minutes apart. It was finished in perfect timing for him to get to work. It was a strange day, to say the least.

After all that, the tests result were negative; nothing was wrong or out of place. It showed nothing unusual! That's good and bad as far as I'm concerned. Bad because I still don't know – nobody knows – *what is the cause of this pain*!

Personal research lead to me to ingest five capsules of Vitamin E, two capsules of Evening Primrose Oil, and another two of White Oak Bark. Drinking Aloe Vera Juice, readily available in gallon jugs at health food stores, is another natural substance. It tastes terrible but its benefits are just that – beneficial – for a persons' immune system. When first reading about the beneficial qualities that aloe vera supplies to a person's immune system, I started boiling it myself. Yes, it grew in my garden as an attractive cactus, and I knew its benefits for burns and used it for first aid antiseptic spot touching, but when I learned about ingesting it, well, include me in!

Retracing this story to searching for a knowledgeable and helpful physician, I was told at UC Davis "to find my own endocrinologist. There are none here." That took place on a visit with Dr. Allen T. back in February, 2008. It wasn't he that said that to me. It was a Dr. O', an attending physician whom he invited into the exam room due to my insulin pump being an AccuChek Spirit. I was under the distinct impression that being an AccuChek Spirit user was a problem – for them. No one there, at that time, was familiar with its usage. We're talking 2007. Again, I felt faced with a bunch of ignoramuses. Such a search without a doctor's specific reference is time-consuming and had left me in a panic to make a choice in order to get prescriptions. Once done, this cycle of "care misuse," I'll call it, starts all over again.

One endocrinologist whom I was acquainted with for many years would always tell me to "lose weight." Okay fine. I could afford to lose ten pounds. Give me the tools, give me the encouragement, refer me to a class of sorts, or something along those lines to accomplish this goal. Refer me to a nutritionist, a dietician. It never happened. I haven't seen or been directed to see a nutritionist since moving to California. That's 20 years now! My weight was and is not a dire issue to me. At 5' 5" 150 pounds, this has been sustained since I was 18 years old. Bite me!

When asked why my HbA1C wasn't where *he* wanted it to be, it was my fault for not doing something right. Always my fault.

You know, as an attractive middle-aged woman with diabetes, I am delighted to say that I have all my original parts except my appendix and my virginity. I think that doctors look at me, think I'm doing just fine, and discontinue their approach to betterment, to positive progression. I have been under the very strong impression that leaving well enough alone is just fine. Yes, I am an expert, *the* expert about myself. I know what I have to do on a day-to-day basis. However, there is no progression *with them*. Thus, boredom. Thus, loss of hope. All in all, my high hopes, expectations, lead to disappointments. I'll never go back! I remain being my own physician.

I am bored with this disease. I have been for too many years and realized this many years ago. I'm tired of it. I want a cure. With this statement, I have come to the conclusion that medical doctors have the same attitude. Many times throughout a person's life, your thoughts, beliefs, values, etc. are reflected, mirrored, with others. Words may never be spoken toward individual feelings, opinions or attitudes, but I've spiritually and intuitively witnessed this. It's one of my many theories. I believe it happens with friends and lovers as well. People have trouble communicating – receiving or giving, listening or hearing – and, therefore, can't express themselves. The words aren't there. For instance, how do you tell a doctor that he/she shouldn't be in this business of medicine because there is no understanding of the patient? There may be a hint of an appreciation for the patient, but no understanding.

Sure, I want the kind of cure that looks to be a liquid in a bottle similar to the size of an insulin bottle. I want to be able to inject myself with it, once and for all, and be done with it. Sound like a dream? Well, it is a dream, my dream. It would be celebratory to give myself one last injection for the rest of my life, no matter the length.

My Diabetic Soul

I did end up locating an endocrinologist, a female, as preferred, and quite unusual, Dr. Adeela A. This tall, thin, olive-skinned beautiful woman has the most gorgeous head of hair! Her personality reeks of gentle, genuine sympathy with a listening factor that has outweighed many doctors I have met. I was happy just to have met her as a woman!

Having practiced endocrinology for four years at the time we met, she seemed exceptionally interested in me. But, they all do – at first. When I complained to her about my so-called "spleen pain" and the processes I had already gone through, she was stumped. She also told me to find a "General Practitioner." "Great," I thought. "Just what I need, another doctor."

The doctor I did finally locate was another chiropractor, Dr. Michael S. In my experiences with chiropractors, they love to cater to people, to whole-heartedly listen to people. The best fact is that I never had had to wait six or eight weeks to see one. My visits have always been scheduled immediately.

After reviewing the X-rays of my spine that I provided, Dr. Michael S. told me the adjustments he would be making. This would require my meeting with him three times a week. That would not be a problem for me if I was serious about ridding myself of this particular pain. The expense of a co-pay would have to be manipulated as with anything else desired. You know, 'rob Peter to pay Paul." Dr. S. suggested that the pain *could be* due to a pulled abdominal muscle with a fractured cartilage located in the area of the rib where the pain was most persistent and insistent. My mind was actually put at ease thinking that this is curable as opposed to having a gastrointestinal complication.

On a pain scale of 1 – 10, with 10 being the worst, I walked into Dr. S.' office with an *eight*. During the course of my visits over a two-week period, twice a week, the pain subsided altogether with occasional bouts no stronger than a 2. My "therapy" with Dr. S., although incomplete at this writing, has been successful as far as I am concerned.

This particular pain increases when my blood sugar levels are too high or too low. I have since taken the pain occurrence as a sign to check my blood glucose level and attend to it immediately. Once again, this disease is a constant battle.

With Dr. Adeela A.'s and her office attendants' help, a General Practitioner was located and contacted immediately. Through overhearing a telephone conversation, it was concluded that this particular General Practitioner, Dr. Jude W., could not see me for another month. Well, I didn't have a month to continue living with this persistent lower-rib pain.

My persistence paid off, once again. Repeatedly contacting Dr. A.'s office by phone, I finally ended up with an appointment – in two days! How wonderful is that.

To make a long story short, Dr. W. ordered more X-rays of the area. They showed nothing. Stumped again, I am at a loss. With no referring physicians mentioned or other possible tests to be had, I left his office with my tail between my legs. I am really starting to think that *they* think I am a hypochondriac!

No, dear reader, this circumstance does not stop here. More doctors – fourteen at today's count – are baffled. This pain remains persistent. I hope to share the cause as well as the cure with you. In the meantime, I remain baffled. Having been diabetic for so long, I thought and hoped that more medical attention would be given to me in this situation. Perhaps the medical society, the medical field, the medical establishment itself would want to help me, to give me more time to live without pain. Do the participants – doctors and physicians - not have a sense of pride?! Boy, am I naïve! I thought I would be special, that one doctor or another would help me rid of this pain. Nope.

This distinct pain is with me every day; I work with it and through it, accomplishing daily tasks as usual.

Chapter 20
We are natural, after all.

An interest in naturalism through gardening has brought my extended reading interests to herbs, their uses, their proper growing needs, and especially for herbs' minor medicinal purposes. This not only has become quite another delightful hobby of mine over a period of many years, but has developed into quite a trend.

Initially inspired by an acquaintance, Patty E., who gave me some of her over-gown peppermint, I rooted it, planted it, cared for it, and watched it grow in leaps and bounds. The scent alone, wafting through my kitchen window, was all I needed to get started. Encouraged, I searched retailers for other herbs and found many. Presently I sow a separate herb garden from my vegetable garden and reap and share the harvest. I use all of them in teas, potpourri, bathing and cooking for healthful consequences.

Further inspired through an infomercial by author, I have read and used the information provided by his writings that pertain specifically to herbs. These books have encouraged my growing and harvesting of fennel "...which soothes the intestines and stomach to reduce gas pains and that bloated feeling." Yes, fennel has assisted in easing this "spleen pain" if only to further prove to me that natural remedies do not get the [medical] attention they deserve.

Digging up my collection of *Diabetes Interview* magazines, there is an enlightening article in the December 2003 Issue 137 written by Daniel Trecroci entitled *"How Herbs and Vitamins May Benefit Your Health."* This article not only encouraged me into this trend of natural healing and awareness, but further encouraged my incorporation of fresh herbs and herbal supplements into my households' diet. Through research, I have come across article after article, book after book, written by different authors in different parts of the world, writing of the benefits of the same and similar herbs. I've been amazed. Therefore, my doubts have weaned to the point of my growing my own herbs along with a vegetable garden. It is cost-effective and rewarding in more ways than one.

Not all the herbs I grow are for managing my diabetes. Some I grow because of their scents; others I grow for a loved one who suffers with ringing in the ears; another who has acne problems; a friend with allergies; stomach ailments; still others because of their tastes and aromas. I use them like spices and with spices. I dehydrate all of them, storing them in glass jars in a special cabinet in my kitchen. You might think I was a witch of old. In fact, through my readings I have come to the theory that many of the men and women that were accused` of witch craft back in the 15th and 16th centuries were actually natural healers through their use of herbs. The useful similarities with wild plants are analogous to our American Indians – helpful and remedial.

Another example is the eating of parsley with garlic. These, together, are supposedly helpful for acne and skin maintenance. You would have to do your own research. I must remind you that I am not a medical personality in any way shape or form! If interested, it is up to you, as always, to research such topics for yourself and others. Another example is the use of Fennel. For me, fennel has become a favorite herb tea. Its natural qualities have truly gotten rid of my stomach upsets. Used with the Stevia plants that I grow and dehydrate, Stevia is a natural sweetener and it has a light and licorice-y flavor as mentioned earlier.

Using herbs as positivity in diabetics is fairly new, but it is familiar to the medical arena. I learned this from my daughter.

Due to Heather working as a Shushi chef, she was able to serve, meet, as well as converse with quite a few different personalities. She has met people from all over the world in all walks of life along with a few 'leading ladies and men.'

On one particular instance of great interest to me, she met Dr. Jerry Gerson, M. D. She was soooo excited that I meet him, she arranged for he and I to meet at the restaurant one evening while she worked. Dr. G. has been a diabetes specialist for approximately 40 years now. His story is his own, but from what I learned after meeting him, he came across an *"Indian herbal formula that has given millions of people with blood sugar problems hope and help."* How's that for an introduction?

I was on to something here, but I remained skeptical. Wasn't this what I was peddling with in my own garden? Heather sure knew how to call this shot!

In respect to Dr. Jerry G.'s research and findings, I think it only proper to share with you, dear reader, a minimal blurb of my internet findings regarding this man and his work. For your convenience, there is a 9-page report, dated 2000, available for your viewing interest at www.diabeteshealth.com. Entitled *Pancreas Tonic Looks for Credibility From Mainstream Diabetes Community*, this brief yet detailed article includes certain legalities involved; pharmaceutical involvement/non-involvement; Ayurvedic Medicine (natural, holistic healing and prevention; read *A beginner's Introduction to Ayurvedic Medicine The science of natural healing and prevention through individualized therapies*); the involvement of test animals (rats, as usual); the people that Dr. G. has met, shared his findings, and encouraged the inspiration for the sale of 'Pancreas Tonic' in the United States; how, due to this particular research, Eastern medicinal techniques have met Western medical techniques and credibly coincide for the betterment of mankind.

Dr. G.'s report is in article form in the Journal of Longevity magazine, entitled *Amazing Herbs Balance Blood Sugar*, dated 2001 (www.journaloflongevity.com). This brief Journal article quotes: "This formula has the entire medical community talking about its ability to normalize blood sugar." This particular article notes eight specific herbs as ingredients, how they are synergized, and some historical facts, and what benefits each herb provides.

Personally, through reading these reports, I not only found them to be intensely interesting, but I also felt quite encouraged. There is a hopeful link through naturalism! It sounds simple; however, I have not, at this writing, invested in a bottle of the tonic.

After being told to "eat a low-protein diet," I instantly found *soy milk*. Not a big milk drinker, cartons of soy is available for purchase in 32 fluid ounce cardboard containers. They certainly do not take up a lot of room in a refrigerator or on my pantry shelf. Made from soybeans, this is another natural resource to my naturalistic lifestyle! It took me a little while to develop a taste for this type of milk after having drank the typical pasteurized/homogenized two percent fat cows' milk for decades. That stuff is for calves, not humans! I mostly use soy milk in my coffee tinctured with cinnamon. Cinnamon is especially good for the circulatory system. Occasionally I will indulge in having a four ounce glass of it. It has a thick consistency to it, and I cannot drink it quickly, but savor the flavor.

As far as purchasing supplements (aka: Vitamins), I prefer those with writing on the label to be a "Natural Source" made with "Certified Organic" ingredients. From Vitamin A through the gamut of so many other supplements throughout the English alphabet, I've used them at one time or another. I can attest to their wondrous qualities. When I've used up one, I'll try something new. Usually I go back to my original purchase. For instance, I'm never without Vitamins E and D and the supplements pycogenol, white willow bark, evening primrose oil, acidophilus, etc.

Read, read, and read some more! Help yourself through research! My constant research into self-help has lead me to these purchases. Many of what I choose to ingest work well with others for one ailment or another. Something for neuropathy, another for retinopathy, circulation, digestion, brain function, menopause, PMS (pre-menstrual syndrome) and a host of uncomfortable and questionable bothers. You need to be resourceful when researching for yourself and your predicaments. Believe in yourself! All this helps me to help myself; it is as simple as that.

My Diabetic Soul

"One of the first conditions of happiness
Is that the link between Man and Nature
Shall not be broken."
~ Leo Tolstoy ~

This is all quite fun, serious fun. I plant, harvest, nurture, and sow vegetables and herbs. I never in a million years thought I would become a gardener. I always seemed such an "old lady" thing to do. I'm not an "old lady" and don't like that stereotype. Someday, I would like to live long enough to be an old lady! Old to me is 85 years of age, when I refuse to drive a car or forget where the moon is located!

Due to my being "retired" from the working world due to Social Security (herein after referred to 'SSI'), sewing, reading, walking, writing, and gardening have occupied my time along with my notary work and its responsibilities. Yes, in summary, I have changed this situation into an envious one, a positive appreciation for life. I am living in blessings of health without monetary wealth.

Not working, however, *not* going to the 9 – 5 office every day, *not* having to sit in a cubicle, *not* having to listen to bosses, *not* having to take care of so many other people and their multitude of accounts with their crises and chaos on a daily basis, *not* having to wake up and dress the part, *not* having to silence my physical and mental anguish in a martyred role, *not* having to hit the glass ceiling – was all quite an adjustment. I finally realized that I was the one to answer to myself. This period of my life was quite an adjustment.

This full-time role as a 'domesticate engineer' has its pros and cons as everything else in life. However, it is life; it is my being able to live as best as I can. Humility had to be re-focused, re-learned along with self-respect and self-discipline. My sense of personal pride was overshadowed by feelings of uselessness. That *had* to change.

Sure, my family is a priority and this became an adjustment for them as well. The now non-existent weekly salary was a big sacrifice. The wardrobe involved with being an "Executive

Assistant" became useless. However, I have kept a few of my better suits for those "just in case" occasions (e.g., a seminar, a wedding, a job interview). Volunteer opportunities abound and I have taken advantage of being able to help others in need.

The knowledge gained from four college degrees has been slowly averted to a 'personal share program.' Be sure to know that just being able to go to college has been a blessing in more ways than one. First of all, the influences and encouragements of such an endeavor encouraged me 'to get a better job.' I did get a better job. I had a number of 'better jobs.' After being laid off for the sixth time – yes, sixth time(!), I initially felt that I had to learn how to take care of everybody else with all their 'p's and q's,' dotting others' 'i's' and crossing their 't's' with proper alphabetization and their scheduling while representing *their* organization. What about me? Me?! I did not graduate college *for them*, I graduated college *for me*!

Through my SSI award, I learned to take care of me, with my holy angelic guides, the gift of intuition, and my acquired knowledge. I believe.

Before getting too far, dear reader, I *must* tell you, admit to you, that I am *not* a slacker. I continue to bring an income into my household, be it ever so humble. I may even be considered as an isolationist because I chose to be an entrepreneur, a sole-and-small business proprietor. This type of operation lent me the opportunity and flexibility to care for myself: frequent doctor's appointments, providing my child the care she required, providing my husband attentions, food planning, etc.

For instance, after gaining an Associate Degree in Paralegal studies, I opened a Legal Document Assistant business. Operating out of my home, I catered to an audience in need of a typist to fill in the blanks of their legal forms. This went on for twelve years beginning in 1995.

My attraction in wanting to gain legal knowledge occurred while having to use the Massachusetts Small Claims Court Division on numerous occasions (e.g., breaches of contracts, assault & battery). I won nine out of ten cases that I brought forward.

After the re-location and settling adjustments in California (detailed explanation in Chapter 23), I thought it would be a good idea to learn about California law. Commuting to college was not new to me, as you know. I rather enjoy it and will continue to feel that way. However, while wetting my appetite with one course of interest, I continued on to another than another, and before I knew it, I resigned to receive a full degree. I'm glad I did!

In addition, I also invested time and money into becoming a California Notary Public. Not only was this service a generalized offering for the convenience of the general public, but it was a greater convenience for my ongoing business and career.

With this subject brought forward, I can' help but share with you a story of a middle age man that I met because of his needing my notarial services.

Initially contacted by a friend of his, his request to me was to drive out to the Napa Valley State Hospital. An approximated 100-mile round trip ensued with his verbal agreement to pay my travel fees of 0.15 per mile as well as the $10.00 signature fee that is the limit in the State of California. The trip was pleasant enough. I brought my usual snacks and juices and waters and cash. I intentionally closed my office, reset my answering service, grabbed my cell phone, and walked out the door.

Upon arrival at this impending and massive ugly grey cinder block institution, I realized it housed criminally insane individuals. I did not expect that! Yes, I thought of turning around and escaping this task, but as a Representative of the State of California, I went forward. After having to go through metal detectors, guards exploring the ins and outs of my brief case, filling out numerous forms, waiting for over an hour, I was finally led into the cafeteria area. Never having met or spoken to the individual who requested my services, a guard pointed "Steven," out to me.

In his mid-to-late 50's, Steven stood at approximately 5'10", with 200 pounds under his belt. Dressed in hospital greens, flat brown moccasin type slippers with an ankle bracelet, he stood when he greeted me and politely waited until I sat. Placing my brief case on a table top, Steven presented the papers he wanted me to notarize. They pertained to his Durable Power of Attorney for Finances. He immediately explained that he wanted this taken care of as soon as possible because he was going to die. "I am diabetic and not doing too well in here," he explained.

Trying not to demonstrate any type of emotion, I examined the pages quietly, lost in my own thoughts. One page required a "witness." Not unusual.

Due to our close proximity to each other as we discussed this matter, a guard came by and told me to move my chair. "What?" I asked dumfounded as he interrupted my train of thought.

"Move your chair!" he loudly exclaimed.

"Move it to where? I'm trying to discuss this paperwork." I harshly replied.

"Ma'am," he said, lowering his voice, "You are sitting too close to the patient. Move to the other side of the table."

I conceded, moving to the other side of the round table that could sit eight people.

Well, my services were never rendered because a witness, specifically Steven's social worker, would not come forth. There was no one else he could ask. I waited three hours for her to show when a message came through, to a guard via a guard stating that "she will be unavailable." I thought Steven was going to cry.

We discussed why he was in there, the horrible conditions, how he never gets his insulin on time, sometimes not at all; he doesn't get any exercise except in his hospital room/cell where he tries to exercise on his own; the food is bad with too many carbohydrates. He looked like a carbohydrate: plump with a yellow grey tinge to his skin, sticky lips that suggested he was extremely thirsty. It was so sad. All in all, the reality of his imprisoned hospitalization brought to my mind the non-regulation of diabetes, the non-existent care. Steven's circumstances really got me wondering, wondering about being a 'jailed diabetic.' With this in mind, all I could do was pray, not just for Steven, but all diabetic inmates and inmates in general.

This experience was an eye-opener, something I **never** want to experience!

Research has always been a requirement throughout my careers. More of a personal necessity than for the service of others, be it customers or bosses, occasions spent at libraries for hours at a time or through the purchases of books, I insisted on learning. For one reason or another, I needed to learn and know the whys, wheres, whats, hows, how-tos, whens and how muches.

Already familiar with operating a business (previously mentioned the typing-for-college-students in 1987), this, essentially, was an expansion of operations through knowledge. Having to keep my net income at a limit of $834.00 a month due to SSI's limiting regulations, I respected that 'rule.' Becoming a Notary Public at the same time also provided me a sense of pride, a sense of being needed and wanted, along with some spending money.

With this being said, such a prospect allowed me to stay home, take care of my family and me. The strategizing of my medication with proper meals and exercise encouraged my non-diabetic and immediate family members. Yes, I have received negative comments and innuendoes concerning my new life situation. Many times, in the company of others, words did not express their exact thoughts. Their gestures, their hints, their insinuations implied something derogatory. I felt it.

"How are you going to survive?" "Is your husband going to have to support you now?"

The owners of these questions, and others, were more concerned with my taking care of my husband, never mind me or our daughter. These certain and few "friends," or so I thought them to be, were totally unaware of or concerned for my benefit. I heard "she did it to herself," or "she's sick because she drinks" or "she's lazy and doesn't want to work." "Why did she get all those degrees if she is not going to work?" Whispers, whispers, whispers.

Greatly, magnanimously, insulted, these untrue comments gave me a new realization of so-called 'friends.' Have you ever heard that you can count your true friends on one hand? Well, I believe it is true. Some people are ignorant with subjective minds. Those individuals I consider to be 'acquaintances,' not 'friends.'

I continue to learn. Such instances further taught me to be humble, appreciative, and more respectful of all life! And, when I have nothing good to say, I don't say anything at all – or I try not to!

I don't need or want such negative comments, or people, in my life. Never once did any of these certain characters ask me how I felt or was feeling. I put such people on my list of those who are 'ignorant of diseases,' not just diabetes. But their lack of compassion, never mind sympathy, will bite them some day. That'll be the day when one or the other comes to me and asks "how did you do it?" "How did you survive?" We'll see. Mark my words!

Through this dramatic change-of-life-through-being-ill, not only do I reap the benefits, but my true friends and family reap as well. Unknown to me at the time I began my first herb garden. Let me explain. This herb gardening endeavor was quite trendy already. After our move to northern California, I discovered that the encouragement of naturalism and holism are extremely popular. I blame it on nature's voluptuous virtues in this area. As opposed to the concrete monstrosities in Los Angeles, trees of all sorts encase acres upon acres of land. There are no trees in Los Angeles County, at least none of significance *to me*. Please remember, dear reader, I am of New England with its plush vegetation, rolling hills of constant green, its colors, and its balance.

In this present and particular continental county, ancient oak trees exist with respect, not allowed to be pummeled and cut up for real estate endeavors. In fact, if a person wanted to cut down an oak tree for whatever reason, a special permit is required, involving bureaucratic paperwork which involves time. Therefore, a person is apt to give up hope of having a certain oak tree disposed of. I respect this with ultimate fascination and regard!

It is healthy to see natures' harmony. It is beautiful. I am blessed to be here with my family. Natural/organic farms are in demand.

My Diabetic Soul

The Napa Valley with its grape cultivators is a tremendous resource not only for the state but the world! This is closest I can get to my beloved New England and its swaths and swaths of forestry.

Gardening is also healthy for the body. Getting dirty, working the soil by hand, always makes me think of Jesus Christ. Even as a little girl, Jesus' attraction to me was felt through toiling in the earth. I do not doubt there is one psalm or another mentioned in the Holy Bible that encourages our species to toil the earth. Well, it stuck in my mind, heart, and soul.

Bending, leaning, reaching, stretching are common body movements when I garden. Without realizing it, my painful peripheral neuropathy has subsided. Exercise, exercise, exercise; positive attitude, attitude, attitude! Not only positive for physical health, gardening encourages the senses of sight, smell, hearing, feeling, and touch. Not only has this activity been a blessing to me and my personal healthcare, I consider a small luxury.

Other inspirations for the use of natural ingredients are the fact that we, as humans, are natural beings. It just makes sense to me.

As a teenager, one of my jobs was a caretaker and a Visiting Nurses' Aide. I purposely became involved with these careers to enhance my knowledge toward my hoped for nursing career. However, whenever I entered the homes of so many patients, there were multitudes of pill bottles all over their homes. It was astoundingly sad to me to know, see, and witness that each person I visited and cared for was trapped into thinking and believing that a man-made, pharmaceutical chemical mixture of toxins was required for them to stay alive. Goodness, if I can't read the words, or understand the ingredients, I won't have anything to do with it!

My sister, Gina, was in that predicament. Unaware of her numerous medications when she was alive, I was astounded and appalled to see the numerous bottles of so many different prescribed pills she had and was taking during the short time before her death. It made sense to me, intuitively, why she was not getting better. She became more and more toxic without relief of pain or betterment and did not realize it, I am sure. I refuse to be put in that situation. I do not want my digestive process to suffer along with my kidney and liver and brain and every other piece of me! I now know better having learned from her illnesses before her untimely death.

Chapter 21
History is the past, present and future.

An irritant to my knowledge and experiences with this disease is the statement "insulin is a cure for diabetes." Such a fallacy! That has been said to my face more times than I can count. As many of you know, insulin is *NOT* a cure. It is a controlling agent to *assist* with the depletion or non-existence of its natural production in a human body. *It is a medicine that has to be taken every day, several times a day, for the rest of a juvenile diabetic's life* <u>*through a syringe*</u>*!*

Author Matt Ridley has it on paper in his book *Genome: The Autobiography of a species in 23 Chapters:* page 249 in my copy reads "...Like the cure for diabetes (injected insulin) or for haemophilia (injected clotting agents)..." To me that written statement is not only an insult, I feel it furthers the death warrant of these diseases. If enough readers believe what is written – the fallacy that insulin is a cure – attentions to a plausible and definite cure will be ignored.

The history of insulin goes back to the early 1920s. "Dr. Frederick Banting and Charles Best are known as the discoverers of insulin. They first extracted insulin from the pancreases of dogs in 1921." **(www.TheHistoryOfInsulin.com and www.Dr.CharlesBanting.com.)**

Ingenuity and desperation were the necessary mothers of this invention, so to speak. As a child, I was often reminded or heard remarks pertaining to the organs of cadaver cows and pigs that were used for their extraction of pancreatic fluids - insulin - for human use. The documented history of this disease amazes me as well as answers some questions. For one, how did people survive? They didn't. How was it detected, diagnosed? How did anyone know what to do? I learned most of this through my research preparation of the yearly Science Fair at St. Mary's. I never won, but I am sure I brought early attention to parents and peers to this disease. That was my sole purpose. It was unpopular in the early 1970's. People didn't seem to care as long as there was 'insulin.'

There is one story I heard of or read about of how a person had to sharpen his/her own needles. How was that done? I have never found an answer and this question will remain in my mind. I am very curious.

There is another story I came across some time ago that I will never forget. During World War I, a highly educated and young husband and wife escaped the harsh European regime at the time. I recall that the wife was 19 years old and a schoolteacher. Although she suspected she was sick, suffering with typical diabetes symptoms, medication was not easily available. Not until they made their own from the cadaver of a cow. To make a long story short, she survived on this concoction until arriving in America where she was able to purchase animal extracted insulin. This full yet short story can be found in an older issue of Diabetes Interview, specifically Issue 114, Volume 11, Number 1 © 2002, page 50, entitled "Eva's Insulin," written by Radha Mclean. It is truly awe-inspiring and worth your research and reading. Interestingly enough, through my research, I also found a substance extracted from, believe it or not, salmon that enhanced insulin that same time period. Amazing.

I have always wondered how it was for many people many, many years ago who suffered with and through the systems and agony of diabetes, even before it was named. I can only think that their lives were short and uncomfortable.

As a "controlled substance, my use of insulin for over fifty years leads me to believe that I am an addict. I have had to use it, I need it, I crave it, I want it. These are the standard physical and emotional strains as with any drug, legal or illegal. Reality check!

Present day "elders" of this disease, whom I prefer to call "champions" are those individuals whom I have only read about that have dealt with diabetes for longer than I. This fact continues to amaze and awe me; to have this disease for 50, 60, 70, and even 80 years is mind-blowing. I'm right there with them if only due to my choice to live while having a strong spirit.

The *Edmonton Protocol*. Ever hear of it? It involves an *Islet Cell Transplantation* as a cure for diabetes. It sounds promising, maybe hopeful, but I've been through such hopeful newspaper headlines.

Featured in an article entitled *"Release from Bondage"* by Elizabeth Cooney of the Worcester [Massachusetts] Telegram & Gazette newspaper, she wrote that "the Edmonton Protocol, named for a 1999 breakthrough at the University of Alberta [Canada] that allowed successful islet cell transplantation for more than one donor pancreas using new anti-rejection medication."

However, the main foci of this particular article are Mrs. Joan Starrett and Mr. Richard Osterfield, "the first two people to receive transplants of islet cells, the insulin-producing tissue missing from the pancreases of Type 1 diabetics." Performed at the University of Massachusetts Medical School (UMASS) facility, [it] "is one of only 14 centers in the United States and 18 in the world offering the transplants to patients selected under strict criteria." I repeat *"offering the transplants to patients selected under strict criteria."* Where does that leave me?

Once again, trying to be hopeful, I collected information and research along with my usual mixture of enthusiasm and excitement after reading through another article written in the March, 2000, *Diabetes Forecast Magazine* by Roger Doughty. And, once again, my personal research was aflame with enthusiasm and hope!

Mr. Doughty's article is so factually awe provoking, I had to read it several times in order to understand and appreciate certain facts. Through intense internet research, I came across the Immune Tolerance Network (ITN – **www.immunetolerance.org**) located in Chicago, IL.

An internet article featured at the ITN website and dated September 4, 2000, featuring Dr. James Shapiro, briefly explained that he "and his colleagues in Edmonton [Alberta, Canada] developed the new technique and will lead the investigation in cooperation with investigators from other institutions. Under his direction, the ITN plans to complete at least 40 new transplants over the coming 18 months in order to further assess the effectiveness of the method."

A key paragraph to this article reads: "If you are a Type 1 diabetes patient living in the USA and are interested in participating in the trial, please review the information on this site. Canadian patients should visit the University of Alberta Clinical Islet Transplantation Program website for further information."

Well, my full attention was grabbed. I didn't hesitate to download a specifically designed application, print it specifically for "*The Multicenter Clinical Trial of the Edmonton Protocol for Islet Transplantation,*" fill it out, had it signed by my endocrinologist at the time, Dr. John Tsao in Torrance, California, and submit it, all of it. *It* was quite a package, consisting of four pages. That was back on August 31, 2000.

A letter from Dr. Jeffrey A. Bluestone, Director of the Immune Tolerance Network, arrived at my home, dated October 10, 2000. Briefly, I was thanked "for my interest in the ITN…your referral information has been received and will shortly be considered by the Network research team."

I was elated! I was in, man! I knew it, could feel it. Overflowing with joy, I called everybody.

Finally, a letter dated February 15, 2002, was received from Dr. B. stating "…my sincere appreciation for your interest (blah, blah, blah)…we received thousands of applications (blah, blah, blah)….Unfortunately after thorough review we were not able to include you for further participation in this trial."

Heartbroken, I dropped the ball. I let it go. I haven't heard another word about anything I just shared with you. "They" let the ball deflate. "They" don't care about me. That is how I feel. Let go and let God. I'll continue to take of *my* diabetes.

My Diabetic Soul

Edmonton protocol

*"The **Edmonton Protocol** is a method of implantation of pancreatic islets for the treatment of type 1 diabetes mellitus, specifically "brittle" type 1 diabetics prone to hypoglycemic unawareness. The protocol is named for the islet transplantation group at the University of Alberta in the Canadian city of Edmonton, where the protocol was first devised in the late 1990s."*

Procedure

"The Edmonton Protocol involves isolating islets from a cadaveric donor pancreas using a mixture of enzymes called Liberase™ (Roche). Each recipient receives islets from one to as many as three donors. The islets are infused into the patient's portal vein, and are then kept from being destroyed by the recipient's immune system through the use of two immunosuppressants, sirolimus and tacrolimus as well as a monoclonal antibody drug used in transplant patients called daclizumab." **Special Note:** The Edmonton Protocol is not a cure.

History

"Islet isolation and transplantation was pioneered by Paul Lacy throughout the 1960s. He and Walter Ballinger together were able to restore normoglycaemia in diabetic rats following the transplantation of isolated islets into the rodent's livers. Scientists have not yet successfully translated Dr. Lacy's success in rodents to humans.

"The Edmonton Protocol was primarily developed by Dr James Shapiro (transplant surgeon), Jonathan Lakey Ph.D., Dr Edmond Ryan (endocrinologist), Gregory Korbutt Ph.D., Dr. Ellen Toth, Dr. Garth Warnock, Dr. Norman Kneteman, and Ray Rajotte Ph.D., at the University of Alberta Hospital and the Surgical-Medical Research Institute. The first patient was treated using the Edmonton Protocol in March 1999. The protocol was first published in the New England Journal of Medicine in July 2000.

"The NEJM report was exciting for the diabetes field because all seven patients undergoing the Edmonton Protocol remained insulin-

independent after an average of 12 months."

Current review

"It has recently been reported that of thirty-six patients transplanted, only sixteen (44%) were insulin-independent after one year; ten (28%) had partial graft function after one year; and ten (28%) had complete graft loss after one year. Insulin independence is not usually sustainable in the long term, but the transplanted islets still function enough to provide protection from severe hypoglycemic episodes and unawareness.

"The major problem limiting islet transplantation therapy for type 1 diabetic individuals is the lack of organ donors."

References

[1] Shapiro AMJ, Lakey JRT, Ryan EA, Korbutt GS, Toth E, Warnock GL, Kneteman NM, Rajotte RV. Islet transplantation in seven patients with type 1 diabetes mellitus using a glucocorticoid-free immunosuppressive regimen. N Engl J Med. 2000; 343:230-238.

[2] Saffitz JE, Schmidt RE, McDaniel ML. Dr. Paul Eston Lacy, 1924–2005. American Journal of Pathology. 2005; 167:299-300.

[3] Ryan EA, Paty BW, Senior PA, Bigam D, Alfadhli E, Kneteman NM, Lakey JR, Shapiro AM. Five-year follow-up after clinical islet transplantation. Diabetes. 2005 Jul; 54(7):2060-9.

[4] Sutherland DE, Gruessner RW, Gruessner AC. Pancreas transplantation for treatment of diabetes mellitus. World J Surg. 2001 Apr; 25(4):487-96.

[5] Shapiro AMJ, Ricordi C, Hering BJ et al. International trial of the Edmonton protocol for islet transplantation. N Engl J Med. 2006; 355:1318-1330.

[6] O'Gorman D, Kin T, Murdoch T, Richer B, McGhee-Wilson D, Ryan EA, Shapiro AMJ, Lakey JRT. The standardization of pancreatic donors for islet isolations. Transplantation. 2005 Sep; 80(6):801-806.

Clinical Islet Transplant Program - University of Alberta
(From Wikipedia, the free encyclopedia.)

Everything is science fiction once upon a time. Creativity is the mother of invention.

Now that I've captured your scientific awareness with this disease (or I at least hoped to have caught your attention!), Stem Cell

Research is the latest trend to cure the incurable.

Stem cells, stem cells everywhere; not a one to use.

What are stem cells?

My very first visualization of a stem cell came from my high school and early college days of biology classes. To me at first, stem cells were minute (smaller than the smallest head of the smallest common pin) energy producing energies. Leaving them to my imagination, stem cells are also tan in color. Go figure. Just like the first mentioning of cholesterol, I visualized cholesterol as being green in color. To this day, I truly have no idea what color are either of these organisms. Imagination at play again.

According to the **Wikepedia, free internet encyclopedia**, stem cells are…

"…found in most, if not all, multi-cellular organisms [such as the human animal]. They are characterized by the ability to renew themselves through mitotic (?) cell division and differentiating into a diverse range of specialized cell types. "

That is simple enough for me to understand, but there's more…

"Research in the stem cell field grew out of findings by Canadian scientists Ernest A. McCulloch and James E. Till (credits to them!) in the 1960s." The 1960s?! Oh my gosh! "The two broad types of mammalian stem cells are: **embryonic stem cells** that are isolated from the inner cell mass of blastocytes (?), and **adult stem cells** that are found in adult tissues. In a developing embryo, stem cells can differentiate into all of the specialized embryonic tissues. In adult organisms, stem cells and progenitor cells (?) act as a repair system for the body, replenishing specialized cells, but also maintain the normal turnover of regenerative organs, such as blood, skin or intestinal tissues.

"Stem cells can now be grown and transformed into specialized cells with characteristics consistent with cells of various tissues such as muscles or nerves through cell culture. Highly plastic adult stem cells from a variety of sources, including umbilical cord blood and bone marrow, are routinely used in medical therapies. Embryonic cell lines and autologous (?) embryonic stem cells generated through therapeutic cloning have also been proposed as promising candidates for future therapies." The question marks have been inserted by me, for good reason.

(http://en.wikipedia.org/wik/Stem_cell.)

Phew!

I'm for it; it's as simple as that. Mired in religious, moral, ethical, political, and scientific facts, opinions, as well as beliefs, I'm still for it. Stem Cell transplantation is progress. Yes, sacrifices have to be made as always and throughout life; and again, there are consequences for every action and inaction. This endeavor is a sacrifice for progress, for healing, for cures.

Andrew W. Siegel wrote in *"A Commissioned Paper for the NBAC"* (National Bioethics Advisory Commission):

> *"The principal moral justification for promoting research with human pluripotent (?) stem cells is that such research has the potential to lead to direct health benefits to individuals suffering from disease. Research that identifies the mechanisms controlling cell differentiation would provide the foundation for directed differentiation of pluripotent stem cells to specific cell types. The ability to direct the differentiation of stem cells would, in turn, advance the development of therapies for repairing injuries and pathological processes. The great promise of human stem cell research inspired thirty-three Nobel laureates to voice their support for the research and to lay down the gauntlet against those who oppose it: 'Those who seek to prevent medical advances using stem cells must be held accountable to those who suffer from horrible disease and their families, why such hope should be withheld."*

The question mark is my insertion.

(Edited by Michael Ruse & Chrostopher A. Pynes. The Stem Cell Controversy ©2003.)

I am not a scientist. And I certainly was not familiar with the phrase "pluripotent cells." So, I read another book! Neither am I a medical personnel person at any level. I am intelligent and well educated. I am resourceful and my personal research and readings have led me to the above mentioned book. I find the above quote to be astounding. Polemics.

By the way, the NBAC "was created by President William Jefferson Clinton with Executive Order 12975 on 3 October 1995. The purpose of NBAC was to provide a review of policies and procedures in the area of bioethics. The commission has produced reports on the subjects of cloning and stem cell research. Directed by Harold T. Shapiro, NBAC's charter expired 3 October 2001."

All in all, this is a must-read book. The stem cell opportunity must be learned and respected. Therefore, once again, personal research is highly suggested.

> *"There is nothing that is either good or bad,*
> *but thinking makes it so."*
> ~Shakespeare - Hamlet Act 2, scene 2~

Now, I need to pause for a moment and distinguish the differences between *beta cells*, *islet cells* and *stem cells*. Do I, or any other diabetic, need all of these cells to be cured? Or, is it one or two? I'm confused. So, I do this research for myself as well as you, dear reader.

Through the "Science Projects" held during my early high school years, my entry *always* involved diabetes. Although it seemed to become boring for my viewers every year, the tasks involved were very simple for me. In actuality, year after year, I was trying to bring attention to the facts of this disease: its demonic, slow killing procedures. My gosh, there were three of us, out of five children in the household, that had this disease! One year, the syringe I displayed in my entry had been stolen. I reported it to the school principal and that was the end of that.

To summarize, and as I understand them, the *Islets of Langerhans* produce *hormone-producing cells*. Particular hormone-producing cells known as *Beta cells* (β-cells) produce insulin inside of the *Islets*. Insulin is a hormone. Therefore, my islets don't produce insulin for unknown reasons, many theories. My beta cells are destroyed by an "autoimmune process."

Stem cells would/could be used to regenerate, albeit re-grow, beta cells in the pancreas.

As with the Islets of Langerhans, the transplantation processes would need to be repeated. That requires multiple cadavers. That process, in turn, requires autoimmune suppressants and sequential visits. Autoimmune suppressants are not pretty or kind to the human body. I've seen what they did to my sisters. Bloating, fatigue, loss of appetite, constipation, etc. If the opportunity arose for me to succumb to an Islet transplantation, I do not think I would put myself through all that – in a hospital atmosphere. Just give me a vial of "liquid cure" and be done with it! Like that's really going to happen! It's a nice thought!

During my lifetime to this point, I have experienced eleven presidents! Beginning with Dwight D. Eisenhower (1953 – 1961); then John F. Kennedy (1961 – 1963); onto Lyndon B. Johnson (1963 – 1969); Richard M. Nixon (1969 – 1974); Gerald R. Ford (1974 – 1977); James E. Carter (1977 – 1981); Ronald W. Reagan (1981 – 1989); Geroge H. W. Bush (1989 – 1993); William J. Clinton (1993 – 2001); George W. Bush (2001 – 2009); and finally, Barack H. Obama (2009 – present).

Never having been politically savvy or even greatly interested for the most part, my attentions to politics arose with the subject matter of the United States Federal Government's assistance with medical research, specifically stem cell research. Yes, I have voted year-in-and-year-out. Yes, I have always reviewed what I was voting for, doing my best for State, Country, and Community. Sure, I have opinions and beliefs, but those don't usually get me anywhere except in an argumentative debate! Therefore, I keep my politics and my religion and my salary to myself. I don't like to bicker or debate. It only raises my blood pressure and increases my blood glucose levels.

Federal funding has become a repetitious request for scientific researchers (aka: institutions) to find a cure of anything, especially in a presidential campaign. I'm for it, all of it: the research, the allocation of funds, the encouraging of brainiacs to find a cure of something! I bet too many of our country's highly educated scientific-types are just busting to be given the chance to alchemize a cure!

My impatience and fright of painful complications with death has angered me to the point of canceling yearly contributions toward diabetes research, toward certain and specific organizations that seem to have a great administrative and overhead cost. Feeling that my contributions were spent on personal salaries and personal everything, I could never pinpoint where each dollar, each cent was being spent. It is not easily accessible public information. It has not been easily accessible to my research inquiries.

On the other hand, I wonder how long it took to develop the useful gadgets now popularized and in use to control this disease. *Control* is the key word. Let's see, insulin itself was a big invention; Clinitest Tablets; disposable syringes; insulin pumps; glucose meters; inhaled insulin; various pills, of course; the gluco watch, etc. Without such devices many of us would have died years ago. Realistically, such things may be considered as building blocks toward the higher goal – an actual cure. As an optimist at heart, I have to find a positive rationale while fighting the pharmacological fascists and the corporate regime.

Yes, I have often thought that a cure was available, sitting on a shelf in some high security storage closet. It hasn't been unleashed to the public because the world would go in debt – again!

Now I'm going to take you back in time. Beginning with Dwight D. Eisenhower's appropriations for fiscal 1960.

On August 14, 1959, then **President Eisenhower** approved H. R. 6769 (House of Representatives [Bill #6769]).

"First, with respect to medical research, every American is of course deeply interested in the improvement of health. This interest is reflected in the Administration's progressive record of support for health activities. But there is a limit to the rate at which medical research can grow and yet grow soundly. Appropriations to the National Institute of Health [NIH] have increased fourfold in the last six years. H. R. 6769 would add a further increase from $294 million to $400 million – or 36% in a single year. This increase gives me cause for concern on three grounds..."

This proves to me that since I was born, there were governmental funds being made available for medical research.

Research collected from "*Legislative News, Volume 49. Number 11, A. J. P. M. Page 1548*:

"...H. R. 6769 provides more than $100 million over the 1959 appropriation for the National Institutes of Health [NIH], representing an increase of 26.5 percent."

Between 1959 and 1993, the presidents in office did not have any insightful offerings toward "medical research policies" that I was able to find during my research.

On January 22, 1993, then **President William J. Clinton** declared:

"Today I am directing Secretary of Health and Human Services, Shalala, immediately to lift the moratorium on Federal funding for research involving transplantation of fetal tissue. This moratorium, which was first imposed in 1988 [Ronald W. Reagan's Administration] was extended indefinitely in 1989 despite the recommendation of a blue ribbon National Institute of Health [NIH] advisory panel that it be ended. Five years later, the evidence is overwhelming. The moratorium has dramatically limited the development of possible treatment for millions of individuals who suffer

from serious disorders, including Parkinson's disease, Alzheimer's disease, diabetes, and leukemia. We must let medicine and sciences proceed unencumbered by anti-abortion politics."
(www.presidency.ucsb.edu/ws/index.php?pid=46219 The American President Project: William J. Clinton XLII President of the United States: 1993 – 2001. Remarks on Signing Memorandums on Medical Research and Reproductive Health and an Exchange with Reporter. January 22, 1993.)

Right on Mr. Clinton!
Now onto former President George W. Bush.

"The U. S. President George W. Bush has used his veto power to stop a bill that would have increased federal funding for research on embryonic stem cells (ESCs) on July 19, 2006. The president and other conservatives believe that the morality forbids destroying additional embryos, regardless of the cells' treatment-producing potential. However, the ESC-research supporters believe that the cells' life-saving potential outweighs the misgivings over destruction of in vitro fertilization (IVF) embryos, most of which will be discarded."
(http://www.faqs.org/abstracts/News-opinion-and-commentary/Stem-cell-research-Is-President-Bush-blocking-important-medical-research? Article Abstract.)

Oh my gosh. How heart-breaking is this? There was so much promise emanating from President Clinton's representation only to be shot down by his successor. However, I understand that our 'war on terrorism' is costly and President Bush's top priority for the overall country-at-large. Waiting for scientists to formulate a cure is a big part of my life.

Headlines dated March 9, 2009, re-cap President Barack Obama's views on this highly controversial subject.

> "In what has been interpreted as a direct rebuke of former President George W. Bush, President Obama said today that his administration would make 'scientific decisions based on facts, not ideology.
>
> "The president signed an executive order ending an 8½-year ban on federal funding for embryonic stem cell research, paving the way for a significant amount of federal funds to flow to science."
>
> **Childs, Dan and Stark, Lisa. Obama Reverses Course, Lifts Stem Cell Ban, March 9, 2009.**
> **(http://abcnews.go.com/Health/Politics/story?id.)**

Yeah! That's not the whole article, but it is enough for me to read. It is positive news. Positive news brings hope.

Chapter 22
Am I going crazy or is it me?

Addressing insanity, there is no wonder, at least to me, that insanity is *another* of many complications of diabetes.

When emphasizing, yet simplifying, the definition of diabetes, I have told people that it's a game of strategy. Diabetes is a constant juggling game. A personal list of facts, what I refer to as "game board pieces," would include a daily schedule with a daily diet; a daily exercise regime; doctor's visits of which I am guilty of visiting eight different doctors, repeatedly, at different intervals during any one year; food planning which would include restaurant menu strategizing in itself; insulin amounts; and so much more as you have previously read and have become acquainted with at this point. As a matter of fact, there is a game board available called "Future Focus the Game for Diabetics and Friends."

To backtrack once again, during the years 1991 - 1996, Kaiser Permanente was my, our, healthcare provider through my husband's employer. A visit to my General Practitioner at the time, a beautifully, tall, slim brunette woman originally from Chechnya. Her name escapes me, but I recall her heavy accent. She wished to check my blood sugar right then and there. Mind you, this was supposed to be a regular check-up: meet 'n greet, consult, converse, find out what we're working with and update prescriptions. Through hindsight, I must have been acting or talking strangely. My blood sugar was 34. No wonder. The doctor immediately called her assistant, telling her to bring me some juice and crackers.

"Are you feeling better?" she asked in her heavy accented voice.

"I was feeling fine to begin with. I had no idea, no sign that I was having a reaction," I replied.

"Yes, you were. And it was very low," she said. "34 is *very* low for you, for anyone, to be walking around! You didn't feel anything, anything at all?" she worriedly questioned me. She almost sounded angry in her concern, reminding me of my mother when I was a child.

"No, I didn't," I said. Memories of my mother and my older sister came flooding back to me, stating those same words. "And I drove here. That's scary."

"How long have you been diabetic now?" she asked.

"Too long," I said.

"Yes, and it has effected your brain. You're not being able to detect your lows, such as this, is quite evident. This disease affects your brain as much as it would any other organ in your body." She explained, I half-heard. I didn't want to hear. In my head, I shut off the rest of the conversation. All I remember is "affects your brain." Oh crap.

Due to the above mentioned episode, I started thinking about getting a dog, another dog, specifically to detect my hypo- and hyper- reactions. I have been familiar with dogs. We had a few growing up ("Midnight" and "Morgan"). And after settling in California, we had others ("Max," "Black Dog," "Jamison," and "Money"). Not only have I learned to appreciate their company, dogs have served my life with a greater purposes: exercise companions. If it wasn't for these mutts needing and wanting to be taken for a walk or a run, I would not do it for myself. Instead of having to wait for a human partner to show or not for a walk or run, I have always had a four-legged friend. Exercise is the reason. I don't think I will ever be without a dog!

With that in mind, and little bit of inquisitive research, there was not a specific "diabetes" dog training program available to assist me *at that time*. Through dog-sitting Jamison for ten months one year, this 100 pound, two-year-old chocolate Labrador retriever would voluntarily wake me in the wee hours of numerous mornings. Thinking he needed to go outside, I got out of bed to let him out but he didn't want to "go out." It wasn't until I tested my blood sugar that I realized, time and time again, that my readings were unnaturally and frighteningly low. Jamison woke me because of that fact. He sensed something was wrong and got my attention to fix it. This was stupendous for him to do especially without having been trained! That's when I realized that a trained pooch could be beneficial for me. However, as mentioned, there was no such program for diabetics. Sure, there were and are other "pooch" programs available for persons that are fully disabled (e.g., blind, in a wheelchair, etc., more dramatically challenged than I), but nothing was available for me with my hypoglycemic incidences.

However, and I must shoot ahead many years in this story to share this exciting information with you! I do not know how I came upon this forthcoming and particular information, more than likely through constant internet research, but I came upon an organization called "Dogs-4-Diabetics" (D4D) in 2009. Founded in 2000, D4D purposely trains dogs to detect hypoglycemia, therefore alerting an owner-diabetic to care for his/her situation. It seemed perfect for me. I was open-minded about getting another dog. BUT, the factors that are involved became more and more limiting and I did not go through with it.

For one, the organization is located in Concord, California, 160 miles from home. Secondly, such an excursion would personally require me to stay overnight. That is a cost I presently cannot afford. Another reason, as opposed to an excuse, is my having do this alone. I cannot physically afford to do that. Being out of "my home element" is not conducive to my well-being. There is a tinge of fright at this stage in my life.

Enough said, perhaps it will happen in the future. I have not given up on the desire for this particular assistance with living. Perhaps you are at such a stage and would like more information. If so, check out the Dogs for Diabetics webpage.

Holding a career with its many jobs and responsibilities as well as caring for a family, household chores and most everything else most people have to juggle daily, diabetes has been my priority. It's not easy. Selfish? Perhaps. The choice has been to take care of myself in order to take care of others. Vain? Not so much in a physical sense. I will not take credit for that sin. But vanity with a strong sense of pride is my guilt to self-satisfaction. I think I am amazing for having maintained myself this far especially after experiencing too many young deaths.

This disease, being constantly on and in my mind, is tiring even depressing. It has disallowed me from participating in certain activities as previously mentioned with water sports. It has disallowed me to eat or drink due to consequences. Great forethought with planning is required on a daily basis. Diabetes has tried to dissuade me from traveling. Such an endeavor not only takes great forethought and planning, but determination and energy as well.

As a responsible and mature adult, I am accountable for what I do or do not do. There are consequences for *everything* without having a disease. I am the only one that can take care of me. And only one of these doctors prescribes medicines for my diabetic healthcare. Albeit, endocrinologists. I'm the one to pick and choose who I will see after an initial consultation. I believe that I am my best physician. I am proactive with *my* diabetes.

So, before I get too old, I'll continue to laugh, or at least chuckle, inside my own head. I look forward to becoming eccentric – I like that word – and wear purple skirts with red blouses and black shoes. People will smirk, whisper, and continue to react as people do. Not only do I love to laugh with and at others, I love to laugh at myself.

Such strategic juggling constitutes maneuvering, manipulating, planning, and remembering in order to caring for me each and every day. If I don't take care of me, I can't take care of you, the other people, places and things in my specific little life. And each day is different. Nothing can be dropped – excluded – without something else becoming off-balance. It is rather stringent. It is being "in my element," a comfortable, well known zone of me and myself. I used to think that people in my company were inconsiderate, even disrespectful, for not giving me the courtesy of attention that I required. I could not and cannot force people to appreciate my life. No one but another diabetic can possibly understand what it is to maintain a life with this disease, especially before *the pump*. For instance, eating out with friends constitutes anxiety. Why is it that friends and acquaintances in my open circle of life prefer to eat dinner/supper late, like 7 or 8pm? That's late for me. Through no fault of my own, my usual dinnertime is before 6pm. However, in order to be socially gracious and accommodating, my gears are shifted without a word, no complaints.

Flexibility has become the best buzzword for the pump. Through its use, insulin dosages can be minimalized or maximized depending upon food intake, exercise level and stress. It can also be turned off or placed on "temporary basal rate." This feature I use quite often, especially during hours and hours of yard work. It allows me to lower my basal rate by a certain percentage and lasts up to four hours. When ill and my blood sugar rise, this feature allows me just the opposite – to increase the hourly basal rate by a certain percentage. The percentages I choose are a guess and I use them at my discretion depending upon how long I intend to be active. However, I cannot choose how long I will be sick. That percentage will remain increased until my blood sugars become stabilized and lower.

For example, preparing my daily wardrobe, I have to keep in mind where the pump will be positioned on my body and my clothing. I dress for comfort and the ease of accessibility. Pants with pockets are essential as are shirts, blouses or dresses with easy access to the pump. Once again, I find myself having to go to a public restroom and privately remove an article of clothing in order to access the pump and do what I have to do.

Sleeping, napping or just resting can sometimes be a chore. Imagine, if you can, having to have a needle in your body 24 hours a day, 7 days a week. When in a relaxed state, such as when I am going to sleep, I position myself to the best of my ability in order not to disturb the infusion–needle–site. My efforts have become useless.

Two or three hours later, pain at any needle site always, and nightly, awakes me. I have now conformed to sleeping for no more than 6 hours per night. Yes, I am tired during the day after a night's tossing and turning and have tried to take an afternoon nap only for the site pain to recur. Most days I don't bother napping or resting due to these facts. I am at my wits end on gaining proper sleep.

To intensify this subject only requires your imagination. Think of your daily accomplishments, what you have to do today, tomorrow or next week, what you like to do and what you *would like* to do. Even sprinkle in bits of your dreams. Compound all that with a daily fight, often an argument with yourself. You don't want to do it but you have to just to get home, get to a better place, even a good state of mind. I've had my desperate moments. We all have. To me, this is a fact that is, has been, natural for mental and physical growth, an acceptance to my and your personal lives.

"A desperate disease requires a dangerous remedy."
~ Matt Ridley, *Genome*, 1999 ~

The throes of peri-menopause, menopause, post-menopause, whatever *they* want to call it, hit me upside the head! Thinking back on 'how' I first got to this stage of life I attribute to the continental shift I made back in 1990. This is when I voluntarily moved, essentially re-located, from Massachusetts to California. Being as young as I was, 34, I never suspected menopause to begin its transformations until aged 50 or so. Boy, was I wrong! Naïveté strikes again!

First of all, the anxiety involved with this re-location would have thrown anyone for a loop, I'm sure. Still a single mom at the time, this endeavor cost me time and expense toward a purported better life style. Was anything better than what I already experienced? Well, the adventurer in me was quite delighted with the thought. I was anxious and eager to find out. With the need in my soul for learning along with beating time to conquer and experience anything and everything that I possibly could in this life, I hastened this move. However, deciding to sell off most of our belongings in a 7-room apartment, shipping to California those we decided to keep, selling our beloved vehicle (the 1981 Chevy Cheyenne metallic blue, 6-foot bed, 5-speed on the floor pick-up truck), and leaving my daughter with my mother for 3 months really wore me out, tore me up mentally, more than I realized at the time. My separation from Heather was the worse.

The pivotal decision happened after being laid-off – again – and I was angry. Still young, I earned for betterment for my daughter and I. As a recent graduate of Worcester State, my brain yearned for a more captivating, challenging, audience. The voices in my head at the time screamed *"Get out of Massachusetts!"*

A friend in California, later to become my second husband, encouraged me to leave. Arrangements were made to live with him, find a job, get settled, and send for Heather. The plan in my head was not as simple as it sounded, as it surely could have been. For one, the Massachusetts governmental agencies coincide with certain California governmental agencies. Specifically, the State of California did not respect or honor the Massachusetts Medi-care system of which I was using. So not only did I pile up on medical supplies (insulin and syringes) before leaving Massachusetts and send them out with all my other belongings, but they didn't last for too long. As I did not find a job immediately, my mother and sister were on stand-by to send me insulin and syringes through the mail. They wanted this life to work for me. They encouraged me 'to go West young woman.'

I had to find a job – with medical benefits – and fast!

And I did! However, it was through another "temp agency." Temp agencies do not supply benefits of any sort unless you have worked for them for a limit of 18 months. I didn't have that long.

With this tremendous concern, my friend proposed marriage. After three months of living with him, I accepted. Believing that he was learning about and experiencing me with my diabetes was another challenge. That process actually took quite a few years. Of course, I had to admit and realize that he could not read my mind when I needed help. Gosh, it is true that relationships take a lot of work. But first, there is the relationship a person has with his or her self. I had enough confidence and trust to make this one work. I believed in myself. Not only would this marriage provide me with necessary medical insurance as a spouse through his employer, but my daughter needed a full time father. I needed to get her out here, with me. I burdened my mother enough.

And so it was. Dreams came true and prayers were answered. I saved up enough money to purchase a 1984 Volvo through my fiancées' cousin on a personal payment plan. Heather was enrolled in a nearby parochial school a mile and a half from this 'new home.' Our wedding took place in La Jolla, California, on my birthday, because that was the soonest date we could schedule the chapel and the preacher. Typical wedding plans were made: Rhonda Cadwell was my Maid-of-Honor. Without her help I would have been at a loss, a great loss, as far as finding 'deals,' places, a florist, wedding-cake-baker, invitations, etc. Her husband, Matt, my fiancées' best friend, stood as the 'best man;' their daughter, Michelle, was the ring bearer. Heather walked me down the aisle.

To conclude, this ceremony was a humble affair. Nothing compared to the event of my first marriage. Guests were all inclusive of my new husbands' friends and family. The only family representing me was my daughter. No honeymoon except for a day trip to the San Diego Zoo in order to have a days' fun with 'our' daughter.

During all this new-life-commotion and upheaval, (the plans, the daily job, the daily house chores, the daily responsibilities, child care, etc.), I never let on that my blood sugars were out of control. My regimented diet became non-existent, my alcohol use increased, the tension of decisions was profound. I never told anybody, but myself. I literally spoke to myself; I had to stop and discipline myself on what I was doing and not doing in order to get back in control, to be the best at what I could do. Nobody knew about this. I did it, alone.

Through this second marriage, we were all enrolled in a common

HMO (Health Maintenance Organization) that was mentioned in Chapter 17. It has since gained tremendous popularity. As one particular medical campus was located two miles from home, this was a most agreeable arrangement. One thing I did not particularly care for was the constant change in attending physicians. I found the constant transition of doctors/physicians with their rapid turn-over rate to be quite unsettling. Once I became comfortable with a medical persona, either for myself or my daughter, he or she would no longer be available and we would have to visit with whoever took their place.

It also seemed limited in its progressive care and its overall care. As I previously divulged the limited knowledge about insulin pumps, this limited scenario continued with every so-called specialist. I found it uncomfortable and tiresome when trying to learn specifics about particular health issues for me and my family members.

Because medical care was an immediate necessity at the time (1991), it took me time to learn of other options that were and are offered. Six years with that particular HMO constituted our family to peruse something known as a PPO (Preferred Provider Organization). Having gone through the *chaotic* medical care of that HMO's offerings, *change* to PPO care has been most agreeable.

Chapter 23
Calling all hormones!

My suspicions of an infamous menopausal stage of life arrived with unrelenting fatigue, extreme and distracting moodiness, with horrible, mattress-soaking night sweats and elevated blood sugars. Awful. Tremendously awful! Frightening! Awaking tired after 6 – 7 hours of a deep sleep each night just did not make sense. That was not me.

My elevated blood sugar levels would begin with the onset of menstruation. This was something new. I consider this as another warning sign that something in my body just was not right. By 'onset,' of menstruation, I mean 'PMS' (self-diagnosed Premenstrual Syndrome). Menstruation is already bad enough without PMS which is the worst. It's uncomfortable and useless. Being "unbalanced" is uncomfortable physically and mentally.

Notifying doctors (plural) of my discomfort and unease, one told me to "take the covers off your bed. You're too young to be going through menopause." I was 35 years old. I still consider that statement to be a lavishly stupid and ignorant remark. Uncaring. The night sweats were so bad that I sweat through the mattress pad and got into the habit of sleeping with a dry, cotton t-shirt on my nightstand each night, ready to expel the wet one when I awoke! I'm talking wet as in wringing wet, not dampened. This went on for many years off and on.

As for the elevated blood sugar levels, I experienced highs of 400 without any other reason. Through research once again, I narrowed down the facts for myself and my endocrinologist, believing that sticking to the facts was all the proof I needed in order to get some type of attention, some type of help in this stage of life. It didn't happen. Let me explain.

When telling my particular endocrinologist that "I have to use more insulin to punch out these frighteningly high blood sugars," he replied "go ahead and punch them out." Once again, I was astounded at that reply if only because I wanted him to order me lab tests to find the cause, the factual cause. He did not. I continued to increase my insulin, especially before meal boluses. For example, eating an apple would cost me 8 units as opposed to 4. Again, I was afraid to eat.

Once these "periods" were over, my blood sugars would drastically plummet to 56 or 38 and the like. Because such instances occurred in the wee hours of any morning (anywhere from 2:00am to 4:30am), I lowered my basal rates for those times of day. My energy level increased and I would feel good. Feeling good to me is being able to accomplish all kinds of things! And I would.

After 4 days of this so-called PMS, it would begin again, lasting for 15 days with spotting, then five days of a heavy flow, followed with another 8 - 10 days of spotting. Heck, I should have bought stock in *Carefree Panty Shields* way back when, but I didn't know. If only I knew then what I know now...Also, and rather intriguing to me, is my craving for chocolate. That was crazy because I could never have chocolate. Sure, I cheated and occasionally had chocolate. There were more than a few times while I was grocery shopping that a low blood sugar reaction would overtake me and the first thing I reached for was a candy bar. Silly, I know, when I could have and should have reached for a juice bottle, but I did not. My candy bar of choice, oddly enough, was and is a *Butterfinger*. Thank goodness I do not type the *M*s on *M & M*s because there would be no *M & M*s! Such instances are my excuse to cheat. Mm, mm, mm.

Through my dubious calculations and programming of my blood sugars and insulin use, I would have three-to-four "good" days. "Good" days for me are the maintenance of a blood sugar level no higher than 185, no lower than 75.

Through my persistence, my research, and a few more visits with my endocrinologist, I continued to list the facts for him along with the uncomfortable symptoms I continued to experience which led me to believe I was menopausal. Finally, he submitted to my having a hormonal blood test. Days and days went by without hearing from his office in reference to this specific 'hormone test.' Once again, I telephoned for results. The results were important to me, very important.

"In order for you to get test results from the doctor," I was told by his receptionist, "you'll have to make an appointment." That meant waiting for weeks and having to pay another co-pay.

Is that right? Is that proper? I don't feel it is, but I put up with it. What choice does a person have? I feel that I was being robbed through the doctors' use of my health insurance.

Nonetheless, the test results were inconclusive. "You're too young to be going through this" the doctor told me. That was a pretty stupid thing to say when it is a well known fact that women have experienced this onslaught at a much younger age. Now I was in my early 40's and this 'imbalance' I'll call was persistent.

"Well," I began to tell myself, "it is time to find another specialist." I did. During our initial consultation, he asked me "What age did you start menstruating." "I was 15," I replied. Hmm, I did not know what that had to do with anything and I let it go. This particular gynecologist ordered the same blood test; we received the same results. "On a scale of 1 to 20 with a higher number detecting an estrogen imbalance, you are at a three," he told me. Well then, what the hell was going on?

Not knowing what else to do, I let it go, took care of myself, by myself as best I could once again. I read up on the subject, learned of herbs that I never heard of before, starting growing some of my own, made lots of different teas and drank them.

My theory is that while hormones are responsible for the regulation of all activities of all organs (e.g., insulin in the pancreas, steroids for respiratory disorders, testosterone for testes health, progesterone and estrogen for ovarian and adrenal gland health), and my insulin not being naturally produced in my body, the effects of this missing link on other hormones is disastrous. If my research is correct, there are 56 hormones in the human body. Astronomical!

And all these critters are running around, floating around, or supposed to be, trying to maintain the human system properly. When something is missing in an operating system as that of a human body, like a missing link in a bike chain, it can become useless. That's called sickness and disease.

In researching this subject, menopause and diabetes, I found that there is, in fact no research, "no comparable data for Type 1 diabetic women. This confirms the importance of future prospective studies of menopause transition among this population." **(www.DiabetesLifestyle.com.)**

This quote brings me back to my negative thoughts on research and spending. They have not come too far together – not far enough for me!

Through the natural processes of menopause and aging, I have become sensitized to many of life's assets, physically and mentally. Limitations to my former abilities have surfaced, as expected, but unwanted just the same. I have become aggravated with myself. For instance, when needing to clear my garden from autumn leaves, I can no longer spend a whole day doing so. Or when cutting and piling wood for the winter, I have become limited to a few hours of such labor. The same goes for working on my car, or beginning any lengthy project. I have since learned to pace myself whereas I used to go like a bat out of hell to get something done.

In my $15^{th\pm}$ year of this phase of life, there was a time, six months to be exact, when I thought I was done with 'periods.' I rejoiced! Already having had an infected ovary removal (oopherectomy), I was told that a hysterectomy was possible in the future. At this writing, ten years have passed since I heard that statement and I have not had to withstand a hysterectomy. However, the symptoms of PMS worsened: moodiness, irritability, crazy blood sugars, etc. These symptoms make sense to me if I was not menstruating. So, off to another gynecologist. This time I insisted on finding a female gynecologist which took me a purposeful and lengthy time to locate.

Meeting each other for the initial consultation, I found this young woman to be an absolute delight! Beautifully delicate, she did not seem to be older than my daughter. A beautiful red-head with a pale, impeccable complexion, she held an air of confidence and higher-than-usual intelligence. Intuition told me that she would help me deal with my concerns, that I was not "just another older woman going through a typically uncomfortable phase of life." I liked her immediately.

More blood tests were ordered: one for endometriosis: all was clear, negative. Other tests were conducted for various reproductive cancers: also negative. She did, indeed, conclude that my estrogen level(s) were very low. Concurring with my endocrinologist, another woman physician/doctor (Hurrah! because they are few and far between), I was given estrogen patches.

With self-confidence under my belt and a belief in what these women advised, I began using the estrogen patches. Between March 17th and May 30th of that year, I bled constantly. There's no delicate way of saying that, or writing it either. That experience was awful! I took myself off these estrogen patches and stopped bleeding within two days.

The heck with that!

Now, having shared with you my horrors of this phase of life, as an optimist I can truly say that I am glad to have been there. I am glad to have had the opportunity to experience it. Heck, I could be dead, remember? Whatever I go through is a blessing. It may not seem that way at the time, but hindsight usually changes my attitude into one of gratitude. I conceded this thought to my original issues of menopause.

I refused pills and surgical procedures. I treated myself through my personal library and to natural calmers (e. g., Kava Kava, Valerin) so to speak. This is not something that just gets healed. I have to grow through it, as any phase of life. It is frustrating because it is so long. And it is long because it takes diabetics up to 5 times longer 'to heal' than non-diabetics. That is another nasty catch to this disease. Mathematically, and in my calculations, my life-phase of menopause will end soon but not soon enough! According to singer/songwriter Jim Croce, *"Time is in a bottle."* Or, it could be if you choose to go that route, with pills being time, I mean.

Often referred to as "the change," or "the change in/of life," there were drastic changes with my diabetes that caused drastic changes with my mind and body. For instance, my body signs for insulin reactions (hypoglycemia) and highs (hyperglycemia) became mismatched: distinctions of lows that normally were equated by sweating, shaking, headache, numb tongue, and/or numb lower jaw line also mimicked highs. Too many times I thought I was experiencing a high through a certain body signal when it was just the opposite. After giving myself a bolus, I would plummet, unexpectedly, into a low blood sugar reaction. You see, my body signs were mixed up: the heavy thirst that accompanies a high blood sugar would exist along with a headache, a sensitivity that could develop into anger, and a refusal to eat.

With all this confusion going on, I became adamant in testing my blood sugar. That process occurred six-to-eight times a day!

The mentioning of a hysterectomy to me is so overwhelmingly stupefying that I cannot express myself thoroughly. It seems to me that when a specialist physician/doctor is also a surgeon, that's what they want to do: cut something out, eradicate a piece or two, and be done with it. Symptomatic as I may have been off and on in my life, I prefer to find, locate, the distinct cause of my discomfort.

Surgery is not unfamiliar to me. My first surgery was in 1969 for appendicitis. After tumbling head-over-heels sliding down Suicide Hill, with the sled landing on my butt, the specific abdominal pain got worse and worse. Off to the Emergency Room we go!

After about four days in the hospital (Saint Vincent's Hospital at the time in Worcester, Massachusetts) beginning on Palm Sunday, my appendix was removed. I asked my doctor "what is an appendix for?" He replied that "it's a little sack that holds all the popcorn seeds you swallow." "Hmm," I thought. "I've swallowed lots of those and better not do it anymore because now I don't have anything to hold them in!"

My mother came to visit me every day. Uncle Starsz visited me a few times and taught me how to play the solitaire card game that I continue to enjoy. That visit in itself was pretty special because I hardly ever got to see him. I am very fond of that memory.

Through recovering, I began getting lazy with being pampered and having someone else, a medical person, stabilize my blood sugars, I was released. There was no sympathy at home! My mother encouraged me to walk, coaxed me to walk, and finally had to order me to walk outside, to get my circulation flowing. She also told me to make myself cough in order to stretch out the skin around the incision. I did and it worked.

Other surgeries included the aforementioned C-section, both wrists for carpal tunnel syndrome, both thumbs for trigger thumb, both shoulders for my suspicions of "frozen shoulder," another wrist due to the dislocating of three-of-eight bones from a car accident, and a torn meniscus knee muscle due to one of my dogs throwing me to the ground to chase another dog. Stuff happens. My successful Lasik surgery was my choice. It was a good choice.

Through all of these, I have found the recuperation process to be the worse. Therapy has been involved initiating constant exercises. A tight watch on blood sugar levels not only to encourage my healing process, but pain medications always took them off the chart, my acceptable chart for my blood sugars.

Time with patience has to be endured. I have always been an impatient person to begin with, yet being ill helped to teach me that virtue.

As for the self-diagnosis of frozen shoulder, when I mentioned it to various orthopedic specialists/*surgeons*, they never heard of it. I went so far as to bring them magazine article copies and internet print-outs of its existence. Shunned as usual, their diagnosis led to "calcium deposits," and/or painful "bursitis." Once again, I feel I have taught the medical community something else. I do not flatter myself by writing this. It is the truth. I am a pioneer.

Due to unbalanced blood sugars, albeit poor control, I suspected frozen shoulder. This condition claimed both of my shoulders with the chronic and agonizing pain worse on the left than the right, my dominant side. I do not consider either surgery a success. Although it has been five years between each shoulder surgery, I still retain pain in both and cannot move either shoulder to do the back stroke while swimming or scratch my back. My collection of helpful back scratchers is dispersed throughout my house. It's just another thing I live with.

Chapter 24
Another big one!

Looking forward to my 50th birthday, yes, I restate I was *looking forward* to this birthday for many reasons the first being that I am alive. I like being alive; I like my life. Simply said.

However, I received an anonymous e-mail letter right at that happy birthday date that snapped me out of my self-righteousness. Being an open-minded, objective person, I thought I at least appreciated the opposite feeling(s), the negatives that many other people feel about turning 50 years old. Not until I received this letter did I realize the full impact of possible depression.

"I am in denial [with turning 50 years old]. If you cannot relate [to my feelings], save this for a few years [because eventually you will]. I send this in confidence to those who can relate [because of being older than me] or, I believe, will keep this in confidence.

"The good:

• Your granddaughter thinks Grandpa is really old because he has bad knees.

• The same Granddaughter believes you are only turning 20, instead of 50.

• Your eye doctor tells you the deterioration of your eyes significantly slows down after 50.

"The bad:

• "AARP sends you their first 'notice of eligibility.'

• "In an effort to look younger, you once again try contact lenses, but find yourself soliciting advice from [the drug store clerk] about reading glasses from the old lady you are sharing that little mirror with.

• "You ask your Optometrist why glasses are getting smaller if it exaggerates the problem you experience with progressive lenses. He/She blames it on Calvin Klein (fashion versus function).

• "One [contact] lens (left) for distance, one lens (right) for computer work, reading glasses for reading.

• "Driving glasses (since my eyes are not quite understanding which one is supposed to do what), you would wear them for driving, bringing your computer eye up to speed with your distance eye.

• "Both eyes for distance, glasses for computer work, another pair of glasses for reading.

• "My solution: For distance/driving, close right eye. For computer work, close left eye. For reading, hold the reading material further away (which requires longer arms).

• "Your current collection of 'lenses:' Contacts – left eye for distance/driving, right eye for computer work. Reading glasses – one pair for work, one pair for home. Sunglasses – one pair for car, a second pair in the future.

Conclusion – You need 3 eyes: one for distance, one for computer [work], one for reading.

• "The dentist: Your 2 baby teeth (yes, baby teeth) decide it's time to deteriorate, significantly deteriorate. You chip/break the right one 3 times in one week. The dentist builds you a new one and prepares you for an implant.

• "Valentine's Day: You call for reservations at your favorite restaurant. All that is left is a 4:15pm and a 9:15pm [reservation]. You take the 4:15pm slot because 9:15pm is *really late.*'

• "You find yourself sneaking a peek at the Senior Citizen menu wondering when you'll get your discount and how much money you would have saved if you were 55.

• "Your older sister sends a joke that would have been funny a few years ago, but now that you are 50, it's not very funny.

• "Your friends send you multiple 'funny' birthday cards in a relentless pursuit to remind you of your age.

• "Your over-[age of] 50-friends say "Welcome to the dark

side."
• "Instead of plucking your eyebrows to shape them, you find yourself in a relentless search for gray eyebrow hairs and end up having to paint your eyebrows on.

"The Ugly:
• "You start yet another diet because you refuse to start wearing a Muu Muu.
• "While shopping at WalMart, you sneeze and 'leak,' having to abandon your shopping cart full of treasures (e. g., reading glasses). While heading for the exit, you pass all those smiling senior citizens (they are smiling because they too sneeze and leak but are wearing *Depends*).
• "You buy stock in *Depends*, knowing that it will go up.
"Regards, Anonymous."

When first receiving this letter, I was stunned, then sympathetic, then angry. Anger has taken the best part of an emotion regarding this letter. For me, who has seen others suffer with and through diabetes, I am glad to have eyes to see while facing retinopathy and its devastating effects; I am glad that I was adamantly taught to take care of my teeth through fear of gingivitis; I am grateful to have a pair of kidneys that work properly, along with a fully functioning liver; I am grateful that my heart remains healthy at this age, through keeping my cholesterol level acceptable and avoiding heart disease; I also find it most humorous when I laugh and leak or sneeze and leak - I laugh all the harder. This all tells me that: "You are here! You made it this far! You are alive!" I am grateful for what I have and grateful for what I do not have. I also look forward to getting older, always have. I intend to age gracefully, allowing what I have learned about my human body to enhance my years. I want to be proof that what I have done is positive. I wish to inspire others to adopt this attitude. I sincerely want my positive attitude to reflect onto others.

***

My Diabetic Soul

"The most difficult thing – but an essential one – is to love life,
to love it even while one suffers, because life is all.
Life is God, and to love life means to love God."
~ Leo Tolstoy ~

Did you know that after, or at, your 25th, 50th, or even a 75th year *with diabetes* you qualify for a medal? As I joked throughout my life about receiving a medal for accomplishing one task or another, this is no joke. This opportunity is analogous to being an Olympian. Training, strategizing, listening, doing, proving oneself and follow-up are key components to making life work in the world of a diabetic as well as an Olympian trainee.

The 25-year medal program began in 1948. To me, this is quite an historical achievement in two ways: for those people having survived that historical era alone along with surviving diabetes in that time period. It's an honorable and praise-worthy recognition!

Through another article in the *Diabetes Interview* magazine, I telephoned (617) 732-2412 and received an e-mailed application.

How cool is that?!

A medal for being a diabetic. Wow! A medal for being a diabetic for that long that can still see (retinopathy), does not have kidney disease (nephropathy) and/or nerve disease (neuropathy), has all her limbs – in short, for those of us who "have escaped complications which occur in almost all diabetic patients by 30 years duration."

Insulin Resistance was another self-diagnosed factor at this age in my life. "Resistance" is the keyword here. It's similar to becoming immune to insulin as a human body becomes immune to the effects of certain antibiotics. Insulin no longer is able to get into the cells, or the cells reject it, specifically the beta cells in the Islets of Langerhans in the pancreas. I believe that I slowly became sensitive to the action, the purpose, of the insulin I was using. I phrase this occurrence as another "diabetic sickness."

My immediate symptoms and cause for alarm was the fact that my blood sugars became a raging-high-living-nightmare and they remained unmanageable for no apparent reason. That sign again - something is wrong! I'm talking fastings of 350 ±, mid-afternoons of 480 ±. Remember, blood sugar levels, according to "the books," should be kept consistent at 120. That has been impossible for me. 150 is more like it, but even the math answer in this equation was unacceptable.

I continued to wear my beloved insulin pump *and* injected insulin. Although seemingly ludicrous, that is what I was doing. This went on for three weeks. I was injecting in excess of 110 units per day. That's unfathomable and horrid.

Trying to regain composure and remain calm, my analytical mind narrowed down the main variables that were involved: insulin pump and/or insulin.

You see, when I began using the insulin pump fourteen years ago, the initial prescribed insulin for me was *Velosulin*. After approximately three years of using it, a change in my insurance coverage no longer validated Velosulin. Reporting this to my endocrinologist, he prescribed *Novolog*. Both are manufactured with a 'buffer' in them so as not to clog the pump tube. Yes, there is a difference. Velosulin, as with Regular insulin, is shorter acting insulin; it lasts for five-to-eight hours and is best used 30 – 60 minutes <u>before eating</u>. Meal planning is a great necessity when using this type of insulin. Novolog, as with Humalog and Apidra, is a fast-acting insulin meaning that the amount injected peaks within three-to-five hours before more will be needed. That is why they are used with insulin pumps because, as with my Accu-Chek Spirit, a minute amount of insulin (e.g., Basal Rate of 0.8 per hour for 24 hours, divided by 3 minutes, multiplied by 60 minutes) is dispersed every 3 minutes. Phenomenal!

Okay, so now I suspected that the Novolog was no longer working for me. Truthfully, I suspected this too many years ago to count, but I do recall mentioning insulin resistance and asking for a prescription change while under the care of Dr. John T. in Torrance, California. The same request with Dr. Conrad T. of Sacramento,

California, went unheeded as well. Once again, I was fluffed off, given no reply, asked no questions, if only because I believe they did not know what to do! So, I remained on Novolog for 10 ± years. With that being said, I had read somewhere that, to avoid insulin resistance, insulin should be changed at least every 5 years. Well, I was well past that breaking point and nobody would listen to me - again.

This time, I was desperate. I tried to increase my exercises by extending my dog walks, using the stationery bike, etc. My diet consisted mainly of vegetables with few fruits. Protein intake consisted of beans in green salads, baked fish, hardboiled eggs, and sunflower butter. I felt as if I were living in the 1920's wherein that was how best for diabetics to survive. I drank *lots* of water. Carbohydrates were almost completely avoided – I couldn't digest them! Two weeks of diarrhea and nausea was a sign of something. I experienced tiredness, once again, and constant fatigue. My brain was getting foggier and foggier where I couldn't think straight, I couldn't concentrate. My eyes blurred. I was frightened!!

And then I bottomed out. That is the best way to describe what I went through.

The previously mentioned *ginormous* (as in large) Bgs, especially the morning fastings, were completely unacceptable in their repetitions. However, I had to persuade my present doctor that insulin resistance was the culprit. I was losing time – life time! I first mentioned this to her upon our first meeting back in December, 10 months ago. I knew I was losing control back then. She never said anything. She wrote a lot. I talked a lot.

Taking matters into my own hands, I first detached from the pump and used what is known as "the backup" pump. It's the same exact thing, but programmed to be used for 180 days as opposed to the "main" pump. With all the hitch-'em-up details taken care of, I contacted the technical department of my insulin pump company once again. I respectfully needed to notify them of my prolonged concerns in order to trouble-shoot my use of the pump and its functions. I was being rational, analytical, diplomatic and respectful.

Nothing unusual. There was a minute possibility that one operation or another of the pump itself was causing me to be sick because I knew it wasn't me! I knew it was the insulin. My intuition told me. My angels told me. I was resistant. This makes sense to me. I did not make this up.

Inches away from admitting myself into a hospital close to home, Dr. Adeela A. finally conceded and gave me a new insulin – Apidra! After notifying her via facsimile a display of my blood sugar readings over the past two weeks, she telephoned me.

"Andrea? This is Dr. A. Can you come in and get some Apidra insulin? I have it here in my office."

"Oh my gosh, yes," I excitedly replied. "I am soooo glad you called. I can be there in an hour."

"An hour?" she asked. "How far are you from here?"

"Twenty miles," I told her. "If I leave now, I'll be there in 20 – 30 minutes, depending on traffic."

"Okay," she said. "We'll see you then.

Still in my pajamas, I didn't bother to get dressed. I grabbed my pocketbook, car keys, and practically flew out the door!

Once there, I would not leave her office until I refilled my insulin pump cartridge, changed the infusion set and targeted a body spot.

Oh my GOSH! What a delightful difference! Within two hours, my blood sugar went from 351 to 202 and further down to 118. That's great! Not only did my attitude change, my energy levels increased and I was, and am, happy again. I got myself back. Ahh! Such a good thing.

Chapter 25
Many battles have been won,
but the war rages on.

I have come to the conclusion that life is lived in between – in between jobs, in between relationships, in between goals, tasks, ideas, and chaos. Sustenance is a threshold I grasp and have placed among my life's actions or inactions. All of life should be savored, as in being appreciated. *Strategizing* is also an extremely important ingredient on a day-to-day basis when dealing with any illness, never mind a disease. You may already be practicing this compliment and not even know it! Flatter yourself! Accept yourself having been effected, affected and diagnosed; accept your child, or someone you love or just plain know when he or she is diagnosed – with anything! Establishing a relationship with yourself is a tough task, never mind the relationships you have, need or require outside of yourself.

I have God's breath in me – and you do to. His breath grew to self-respect and respect of others. My relationship with myself involves ongoing interactions that contribute to society. Oftentimes silent and alone, interactions are included in the chain of life.

Death can be difficult. It is also expected. I do not want to die in pain, especially pain(s) cause by myself through my diabetes. I do not want to die missing body parts. Too many diabetes complications result in such factors of toe and limb amputations and failure of inner organs requiring a transplant. Unless I take sincere and serious care of myself, death will come sooner than desired. After all, reality of death is the greatest of denials. It causes pain and hardship for our survivors. Surrounded with this reality, I have embraced the depths of much knowledge. Grasping time through knowledge I have been inspired to invest time in myself first and then others that closely surround me.

> *"For death does not end life but is part of it, one of nature's transformations as we work our way through its cycles. Death informs life. It is not, as your poet says, simply the mother of beauty; it is the mother of life itself or how could we conceive of life if there were no death? In addition, it is only because we conceive of life that we know we must taste it lingeringly, try every flavor and nuance, and drink in every experience while we can. Death and life are dependent upon each other, like order and chaos, neither concept being possible without the other. So there should be no fear of death, which is omnipresent, part of life. Welcome it into your arms, for it is but rest: For you lie in nature like a heartbeat."*
>
> ~ William Butler Yeats ~

To know good and goodness does not necessarily mean I will follow it. I know that I am accountable for my well-being as well as you are accountable for your well-being. Consequences, as they come, and they will, are astounding no matter how big or small, no matter how you are affected.

Through the many salaried careers I have held, my most important career has been taking care of myself. The human body is so ridiculously fragile, so unprotected from outside forces, intruders and intrusions. "Taking care" is a phrase to live by, literally and figuratively

I have had to fight for what is truly mine in life: the intangibles such as respect, all emotions, all things learned, all opinions made; and my intangible and ever-present resources. The tangibles include but are not limited to food, clothing and shelter, medication, society. Know it. This book was written to fan the flames of your lives, to inspire you. Know and be known. Help and be helped. Love and be loved. If you are able to read and understand this book, you are not inept. Make it good. Make it all good. Share. Believe in yourself. Be

visceral. And learn then learn some more!
Take care!

References

Further Book, Magazine and Article Reading/Research Resources and Suggestions:

Accu-chek professional's pocket guide to infusion site management. © 2006. Disetronic Medical Systems, Inc., 11800 Exit 5 Parkway, Suite 120, Fishers, Indiana 46037.

American Diabetes Association. Winning with Diabetes, © 1997, American Diabetes Association, 1660 Duke Street, Alexandria, Virginia, 22314.

Baker, Jerry. Herbal Pharmacy1,347Super Secrets for Growing and Using Herbal Remedies, © 2000, American Master Products, Inc., Jerry Baker, P. O. Box 1001, Wixom, Michigan, 48393; http://www.Jerry Baker.com.

Barron, Jon. Lessons From The Miracle Doctors © 1999, distributed by Healing America, Inc.; www, jonbarron.org.

Childs, Dan and Stark, Lisa. Obama Reverses Course, Lifts Stem Cell Ban, March 9, 2009. http://abcnews.go.com/Health/Politics/story?id.

Choquette, Sonia. Ask Your Guides Connecting to Your Divine Support System, © 2006, Hay House, Inc., Carlsbad, CA.

Diabetes Interview (magazine). January, 2001, Issue 102, Volume 10, Number 1; through February, 2004, Issue 139, Volume 13, Number 2; Kings Publishing, Inc., 3715 Balboa Street, San Francisco, CA, 94121.

Dorris, Tamara. Get Well Now! How to Heal and Prevent Disease,

© 2003, Empowered Press   Publishing, 3201 Smathers Way, Suite 2, Carmichael, California, 95608; www.empoweredpress.org.

The Holy Bible Revised Standard Version © 1952; Numbers 21:4-9
Legislative News, Volume 49. Number 11, A. J. P. M. Page 1548, © 1959.

Lund, JoAnna M. The Diabetic's Healthy Exchanges Cookbook, © 1996, The Berkeley Publishing Group, 375 Hudson Street, New York, New York, 10014.

Mclean, Radha. Diabetes Interview, January 2002, Issue 114, Volume 11, Number 1, page 50; Kings Publishing, Inc., 3715 Balboa Street, San Francisco, CA, 94121.

Mayers, Dara. Diabetes Interview, October 2003, Issue 135, Volume 12, Number 10, page 35; Kings Publishing, Inc., 3715 Balboa Street, San Francisco, CA, 94121.

McNutt, Kristen, PhD., JD. Diabetes Interview, February 2004, Issue 139, Volume 13, Number 2, page 38; Kings Publishing, Inc., 3715 Balboa Street, San Francisco, CA, 94121.

Ridley, Matt. The Autobiography of a species in 23 Chapters Genome, © 1999. Harper Collins Publishers, Inc., 10 East 53rd Street, New York, NY, 10022.

Ruse, Michael & Pynes, Christopher A. The Stem Cell Controversy ©2003, Prometheus Books, 59 John Glenn Drive, Amherst, New York 14228-2197.

Shakespeare, William. Hamlet, Act 2, scene 2.
Shanbhag, Vivek, M. D. (Ayurveda, N. D.). A beginner's Introduction to Ayurvedic Medicine The science of natural healing and prevention through individualized therapies; © 1994, Keats

Publishing, Inc., New Canaan, Connecticut.

Sonneborn, Liz. Clara Barton Founder, American Red Cross;© 1992, Chelsea House Publishers, a division of Main Line Book Co.

Sokolowski, Marie and Jasinski, Irene. Treasured Polish Recipes for Americans, © 1948, Polanie Publishing Company, Minneapolis, Minnesota.

Trudeau, Kevin. Natural Cures "They" Don't Want You To Know About, © 2004. Alliance Publishing Group, Inc., P. O. Box 92271, Elk Grove Village, Illinois, 60009.

Trecroci, D. Diabetes Interview, "Here's Glucose in Your Eye," © 2001, Issue 112, Volume 10, Number 13, p. 24; Kings Publishing, Inc., 3715 Balboa Street, San Francisco, CA, 94121.

Wilen, Joan and Wilen, Lydia. Bottom Line's Healing Remedies, © 2007, Bottom Line Books, 281 Tresser Blvd., Stamford, Connecticut 06901.

Internet Reference Resources

www.AndreaDoria.org
http://www.ClaraBartonBirthplace.org
www.DiabetesinControl.com
http://www.diabetes.webmd.com
http://www.faqs.org/abstracts/News-opinion-and-commentary/Stem-cell-research-Is-President-Bush-blocking-important-medical-research? Article Abstract.
www.faqs.org/faqs/diabetes/faq/part2/section-9.html
www.diabeteshealth.com

http://diabetic.healthcentersonline.com
Clinical Islet Transplant Program - University of Alberta.
www.TheHistoryOfInsulin.com
www.Dr.CharlesBanting.com.
www.immunetolerance.org.
http://www.medra.com or medrainc@medra.com.
www.medscape.com.
www.presidency.ucsb.edu/ws/index.php?pid=46219.

The American President Project: William J. Clinton XLII President of the United States: 1993 – 2001. Remarks on Signing Memorandums on Medical Research and Reproductive Health and an Exchange with Reporters. January 22, 1993.

http://en.wikipedia.org/wiki/Elliott_P._Joslin.
(http://en.wikipedia.org/wik/Stem_cell).

Wikipedia, the free encyclopedia.

Dreams are what the world is made of.
Of what is not today, yet possible tomorrow.
Of things unthinkable today,
Yet commonplace tomorrow.
Of problems unsolvable today,
Yet solutions tomorrow.
Of life in poverty today,
Yet riches tomorrow.
You may become only as great as
Your Dreams. "

~ **Michael Wynn** ~

Enjoy a Preview of A. K. Buckroth's next book:

I found him on the kitchen table.
Memoirs

"January 21, 1975

Hi, I'm your dad. Always have and always will be, no doubt about it. It is just that a grown up person doesn't always act grown-up and roots, like those of trees, are torn out like with a bulldozer tractor and if some of the roots remain strong, some day, on some spring day, you might see a bird or two looking for the warmth of the sun.

What I'm trying to say, Andy, is that you, all you kids, have been on my thoughts wherever I go or whatever I do. Your Dad is like a Nomadic wanderer – no real roots anymore, but there are those springtime buds. And it happened – you are the buds, you and Lynn, Alex, Marie, and Louise. I've waited so-oo long for just one bud to flower. It did.

This letter has been written at least 102 times since I heard from you. I don't know why you should be apprehensive writing to me, after all, girl, you carry my name still – and its your right and obligation. Of course this is probably hard to understand after growing up under one-sided impressions.

Let's see, the best picture I have of you, I think your Aunt Marian took in color of a First Communion in from of the house. You were in white, naturally, and your brother, Alex (do you call him that or Buck or what?), was wearing a red jacket and your cousin, Joseph, was standing behind you. I think I still have it secreted away in some of my things.

How many times I've wished to hear you talk to me, ask me questions, tell me what you are doing, how you are feeling. Boy!

I Found Him on the Kitchen Table

And how are you feeling, Andy? I'm sure that you understand about your body and its needs for insulin. It's probably been drilled into you enough. I'm also sure you can sense times when you start to feel woozy and all. Heck, You're a young woman now, I don't have to go into things, do I.

Before I forget about it, I should also say Happy Birthday to you. Let's see, you're about nineteen now, no, no, you are seventeen. Ha! Sweet seventeen and never been kissed? I'll bet you have a whole houseful of boys in every corner, ha ha!

Well, after I left the U. S. in 1965 and volunteered to come here to this hellhole, a lot of water has flowed under the bridge.

In the beginning of our second relationship as daughter-to-father, and vice versa, we met through letters. The first letter is dated 1975.

Not having seen or known this man, my biological father, since the age of 6½, I was now 18. In this writing, not only have I referred to him as "dad," but "Lucky" as well, one of his numerous nicknames.

Being raised and educated through my mother, she greatly influenced me and my immediate siblings. We were raised to believe that our father was "pure evil." Negativity overrode any and all conversations pertaining to his existence. Mothers' rationale was quite contradictory to me at times, especially during my childhood, strengthening a strong misunderstanding of a very young child to her mother. The first contradiction I came to acknowledge was that they were married for twelve years and conceived five children. This is one of many contradictions involving the divorce factor.

I am a creation of the factors.